BLUEPRINTS
Q&A Step 2 Medicine

Second Edition

D0109445

DREXEL UNIVERSITY
HEALTH SCIENCES LIBRARIES
HAHNEMANN LIBRARY

BLUEPRINTS
Q&A Step 2 Medicine

Second Edition

Brenda L. Shinar, MD
Assistant Program Director
Department of Internal Medicine
Banner Good Samaritan Medical Center
Phoenix, Arizona
Clinical Professor of Internal Medicine
University of Arizona College of Medicine
Tucson, Arizona

Series Editor:

Michael S. Clement, MD, FAAP
Mountain Park Health Center
Clinical Lecturer in Family and Community Medicine
University of Arizona College of Medicine
Consultant, Arizona Department of Health Services
Phoenix, Arizona

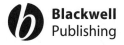

Blackwell
Publishing

© 2005 by Blackwell Publishing

Blackwell Publishing, Inc., 350 Main Street, Malden, Massachusetts 02148-5018, USA
Blackwell Publishing Ltd, 9600 Garsington Road, Oxford OX4 2DQ, UK
Blackwell Publishing Asia Pty Ltd, 550 Swanston Street, Carlton, Victoria 3053, Australia

All rights reserved. No part of this publication may be reproduced in any
form or by any electronic or mechanical means, including information storage
and retrieval systems, without permission in writing from the publisher,
except by a reviewer who may quote brief passages in a review.

04 05 06 07 5 4 3 2 1

ISBN: 1-4051-0389-2

Library of Congress Cataloging-in-Publication Data

   Blueprints Q&A step 2. Medicine.—2nd ed./ [edited by] Brenda L. Shinar.
    p. ; cm.
   Includes index.
   ISBN 1-4051-0389-2 (pbk.)
    1. Medicine—Examinations, questions, etc.   2. Physicians—Licenses—United States—
Examinations—Study guides.   I. Shinar, Brenda L.   II. Title: Blueprints Q and A step 2.
Medicine. III. Title: Medicine.
   [DNLM: 1. Clinical Medicine—Examination Questions.   WB 18.2 B658 2005]
   R834.5.B58 2005
   616′. 0076—dc22

                                2004013543

A catalogue record for this title is available from the British Library

Acquisitions: Nancy Anastasi Duffy
Development: Kate Heinle
Production: Debra Murphy
Cover design: Hannus Design Associates
Interior design: Mary McKeon
Typesetter: TechBooks in New Delhi, India
Printed and bound by Capital City Press in Berlin, VT

**WB
18.2
B658
2005**

For further information on Blackwell Publishing, visit our website:
www.blackwellmedstudent.com

Notice: The indications and dosages of all drugs in this book have
been recommended in the medical literature and conform to the practices of
the general community. The medications described do not necessarily have
specific approval by the Food and Drug Administration for use in the
diseases and dosages for which they are recommended. The package insert for
each drug should be consulted for use and dosage as approved by the FDA.
Because standards for usage change, it is advisable to keep abreast of
revised recommendations, particularly those concerning new drugs.

The publisher's policy is to use permanent paper from mills that operate a sustainable forestry
policy, and which has been manufactured from pulp processed using acid-free and elementary
chlorine-free practices. Furthermore, the publisher ensures that the text paper and cover board
used have met acceptable environmental accreditation standards.

Contents

Contributors

Sarah Beaumont, MD
Chief Resident, Internal Medicine/Pediatrics
Banner Good Samaritan Medical Center
Phoenix Children's Hospital
Phoenix, Arizona

Darren G. Deering, DO
Chief Resident, Department of Internal Medicine/Pediatrics
Banner Good Samaritan Medical Center
Phoenix, Arizona

Tressia Shaw, MD
Chief Resident, Internal Medicine/Pediatrics
Banner Good Samaritan Medical Center
Phoenix Children's Hospital
Phoenix, Arizona

Reviewers

Rodolfo Chinririos, MD
Intern, Internal Medicine
Jackson Memorial Hospital
Miami, Florida

Michael J. Hoffman, Jr.
Class of 2004
Robert Wood Johnson Medical School
University of Medicine and Dentistry of New Jersey
Piscataway, New Jersey

Jennifer W. Lai, MD
Resident, Internal Medicine
Santa Clara Valley Medical Center
San Jose, California

Preface

Thank you! We know that you, our customers, have successfully used the first edition of the *Blueprints* Q&A series to study for Boards and shelf exams. We also learned that those of you in physician assistant, nurse practitioner, and osteopath programs have found the series helpful to review for Boards and rotation exams.

At Blackwell, we think of our customers as our secret weapon. For every book Blackwell publishes, we rely heavily on the opinions of our customers, and we credit much of our success to the feedback we get from you. Your comments, suggestions—even complaints—help determine everything from content to features to the design of our books. The second edition of the *Blueprints* Q&A series is an excellent example of how much influence your feedback truly has:

- You asked for more questions per book, so the questions have doubled (200 per book!).
- You wanted questions that better reflect the format of the Boards, so all questions have been updated to match the curent USMLE format for Step 2.
- You liked the detailed explanations for every answer—right or wrong—so we made sure that complete correct and incorrect answers were provided for each question.
- You needed a smaller trim size for easier portability, and now you have it. This edition is small enough to fit in a white coat pocket.
- You were looking for an easier way to test yourself, and we redesigned this edition to do just that. Answer keys and tabbed sections make for easier navigation between questions and answers.
- You wanted an index for easy reference, and you got it (along with abbreviations and normal lab values).

We hope you like this new edition of the *Blueprints* Q&A series as much as we do. And keep your suggestions and ideas coming! Please send any comments you may have about this book, or any book in the *Blueprints* series, to *blue@bos.blackwellpublishing.com*.

The Publisher
Blackwell Publishing

Acknowledgments

There are many people who helped to make this project a reality. Thank you to my contributors, Darren Deering, Sarah Beaumont, and Tressia Shaw. Thank you to my mentors and colleagues at "Good Sam," Dr. Alan Leibowitz, Dr. Bob Raschke, Dr. Michelle Park, and Dr. Grant Hertel. Thanks to Kate Heinle at Blackwell Publishing for her advice, and to Frank Wallace for his computer genius. Most of all, thanks to my wonderful family for their love, encouragement, and support of my endeavors, and to my husband, Ron, who completes me.

—Brenda

There are several people I would like to thank: first of all, my family, whose love and unwavering support have made me the person I am today; my friends, who put up with me during this project; Sarah and Tressia for being there when the going gets tough; Donna, for having the first faith in me as a physician and as a friend; Barb and Kristin—for *everything* you have done for me through the years; and to "J. Crew" for all the happiness you have brought into my life. This project is dedicated to my parents—words can never repay the gifts that you have given me.

—Darren

First, I would like to thank Brenda Shinar for her guidance in this project. Without the help of my "sisters" Tressia and Doreen, this task would have been impossible. A special thanks goes to Donna for her support, guidance, and friendship. Last but not least, I thank my parents, Matthew, Jackson, and my husband, Doug.

—Sarah

There are many people who have been great influences in my life. I would especially like to thank my wonderful colleagues and friends Sarah, Darren, Donna, and Jodi. Thanks to Brenda Shinar for including me in this project. But most of all, I would like to acknowledge my family—thanks Mom, Dad, and Amy for always believing in me and supporting my endeavors.

—Tressia

Abbreviations

A-a	alveolar-arterial
ABG	arterial blood gas
ACE	angiotensin-converting enzyme
ACTH	adrenocorticotropic hormone
AFB	acid-fast bacillus
AI	aortic insufficiency
AIDS	acquired immunodeficiency syndrome
AIHA	autoimmune hemolytic anemia
ALL	acute lymphocytic leukemia
ALT	alanine aminotransferase
AML	acute myelogenous leukemia
Anti-HBC	antibody to hepatitis B core
AP	anteroposterior
APC	adenomatous polyposis coli
aPTT	activated partial thromboplastin time
AS	aortic stenosis or ankylosing spondylitis
ASCUS	atypical squamous cells of unknown significance
ASD	atrial septal defect
ASO	anti-streptolysin O
AST	aspartate aminotransferase
β-HCG	beta-human chorionic gonadotropin
BMI	body mass index
BP	blood pressure
BPH	benign prostatic hypertrophy
BRBPR	bright red blood per rectum
BRCA-1 and-2	breast cancer gene mutations 1 and 2
BUN	blood urea nitrogen
CAD	coronary artery disease
CAP	community-acquired pneumonia
CHF	congestive heart failure
CLL	chronic lymphocytic leukemia
CML	chronic myelogenous leukemia
CMV	cytomegalovirus
COPD	chronic obstructive pulmonary disease
CPK	creatine phosphokinase
CPK-MB	creatine phosphokinase MB isoenzyme
CPPD	calcium pyrophosphate dihydrate
CT	computerized tomogram
CVA	cerebrovascular accident
DIC	disseminated intravascular coagulation
DIP	distal interphalangeal (joint)
DKA	diabetic ketoacidosis
dL	deciliter
DVT	deep venous thrombosis
EBV	Epstein-Barr virus
ECG	electrocardiogram
EGD	esophagogastroduodenoscopy
ECG	electrocardiogram
ENT	ears, nose, and throat
ER	emergency room
ERCP	endoscopic retrograde cholangiopancreatography
FAP	familial adenomatous polyposis
FEV$_1$	forced expiratory volume in 1 second
FOBT	fecal occult blood testing
FSH	follicle-stimulating hormone
FTA-ABS	fluorescent treponema antibody-absorption
G6PD	glucose 6-phosphate dehydrogenase
GERD	gastroesophageal reflux disease
GI	gastrointestinal
GU	genitourinary
HA	hydroxyapatite
HAART	highly active anti-retroviral therapy
HAV	hepatitis A virus
HBSAb	hepatitis B surface antibody
HBSAg	hepatitis B surface antigen
HCM	hypertrophic cardiomyopathy (also called HOCM)
HCV	hepatitis C virus
HDL	high-density lipoprotein
HEENT	head, eyes, ears, nose, throat

HELLP	hemolysis, elevated liver enzymes, low platelets
HgbA1C	hemoglobin A1C
HHV-8	human herpes virus-8
HIV	human immunodeficiency virus
HMG-CoA	hydroxy-methylglutaryl-coenzyme A
HOCM	hypertrophic obstructive cardiomyopathy
HNPCC	hereditary nonpolyposis colorectal cancer
HPF	high power field
HPV	human papilloma virus
HR	heart rate
HSV	herpes simplex virus
HTLV-1	human T-cell lymphotropic virus-1
HUS	hemolytic uremic syndrome
IBD	inflammatory bowel disease
ICU	intensive care unit
iPTH	intact parathyroid hormone
ITP	idiopathic thrombocytopenic purpura
IUD	intrauterine device
IV	intravenous
IVDA	intravenous drug abuse
IVIG	intravenous immunoglobulin
JNC-VII	joint national commission VII
KUB	kidneys, ureters, bladder (a plain abdominal X-ray)
L	liter
LDH	lactate dehydrogenase
LDL	low density lipoprotein
LH	luteinizing hormone
LVH	left ventricular hypertrophy
MAC	membrane attack complex
MALT	mucosa-associated lymphoid tissue
MCHC	mean corpuscular hemoglobin concentration
MCP	metacarpal-phalangeal (joint)
MCV	mean corpuscular volume
MGUS	monoclonal gammopathy of unknown significance
MHC	major histocompatibility complex
MMSE	Mini-Mental State examination
MTP	metatarsal-phalangeal (joint)
NBT	nitroblue tetrazolium
ng	nanogram
NLD	necrobiosis lipoidica diabeticorum
NPH	normal pressure hydrocephalus
NPO	nil per os (nothing by mouth)
NSAID	nonsteroidal anti-inflammatory drug

OA	osteoarthritis
OCP	oral contraceptive pill
OSA	obstructive sleep apnea
paO_2	partial pressure of O_2 in arterial blood
Pap	Papanicolaou (smear)
PCP	*Pneumocystis carinii* pneumonia
PDA	patent ductus arteriosus
PE	pulmonary embolism
PFT	pulmonary function tests
PID	pelvic inflammatory disease
PIP	proximal interphalangeal (joint)
PMN	polymorphonuclear (white blood cell)
PO	per os (by mouth)
pO_2	oxygen partial pressure
POMC	pro-opiate melanocorticotropin
PPD	purified protein derivative
PT	prothrombin time
PTH	parathyroid hormone
PTH-rP	parathyroid hormone-related peptide
PTT	partial thromboplastin time (same as aPTT)
RA	rheumatoid arthritis
RBC	red blood cell
RDW	red cell distribution width
RF	rheumatoid factor
RPR	rapid plasma reagin
RR	respiratory rate
SCD	sequential compression device
SLE	systemic lupus erythematosus
SPEP	serum protein electrophoresis
STD	sexually transmitted disease
SVC	superior vena cava
TB	tuberculosis
TEE	transesophageal echocardiogram
TP	total protein
TSH	thyroid stimulating hormone
TTE	transthoracic echocardiogram
TTP	thrombotic thrombocytopenic purpura
UPEP	urine protein electrophoresis
UTI	urinary tract infection
VDRL	Venereal Disease Research Laboratory (test)
VLDL	very low density lipoprotein
VSD	ventricular septal defect
VTE	venous thromboembolism
WBC	white blood cell
WPW	Wolff-Parkinson-White syndrome

Normal Ranges of Laboratory Values

U.S. traditional units are followed in parentheses by equivalent values expressed in SI units.

Bloood, Plasma, and Serum Chemistries

Acetoacetate, plasma	<1 mg/dL (0.1 mmol/L)
Alpha-fetoprotein, serum	0–20 ng/mL (0–20 μg/L)
Aminotransferase, alanine (ALT, SGPT)	0–35 U/L
Aminotransferase, aspartate (AST, SGOT)	0–35 U/L
Ammonia, plasma	40–90 μg/dL (23–47 μmol/L)
Amylase, serum	0–130 U/L
Antistreptolysin O titer	<150 units
Ascorbic acid (vitamin C), blood	0.4–1.5 mg/dL (23–86 μmol/L);
leukocyte	<20 mg/dL (<3.5 μmol/L)
Bicarbonate, serum	23–28 mEq/L (23–28 mmol/L)
Bilirubin, serum	
Total	0.3–1.2 mg/dL (5.1–20.5 μmol/L)
Direct	0–0.3 mg/dL (0–5.1 μmol/L)
Blood gases, arterial (room air)	
pO_2	80–100 mmHg
pCO_2	35–45 mmHg
pH	7.38–7.44
Calcium, serum	9–10.5 ng/dL (2.2–2.6 mmol/L)
Carbon dioxide content, serum	23–28 mEq/L (23–28 mmol/L)
Carcinoembryonic antigen	<2 ng/mL (2 μg/L)
Carotene, serum	75–300 μg/dL (1.4–5.6 μmol/L)
Ceruloplasmin, serum	25–43 mg/dL (250–430 mg/L)
Chloride, serum	98–106 mEq/L (98–106 mmol/L)
Cholesterol, total, plasma	150–199 mg/dL (3.88–5.15 mmol/L), desirable
Cholesterol, low-density lipoprotein (LDL), plasma	≤130 mg/dL (3.36 mmol/L), desirable
Cholesterol, high-density lipoprotein (HDL), plasma	≥40 mg/dL (1.04 mmol/L), desirable
Complement, serum	
C3	55–120 mg/dL (550–1200 mg/L)
Total	36–55 U/mL (37–55 kU/L)
Copper, serum	70–155 μg/dL (11.0–24.3 μmol/L)
Creatine kinase, serum	30–170 U/L
Creatinine, serum	0.7–1.3 mg/dL (61.9–115.0 μmol/L)
Delta-aminolevulinic acid, serum	15–23 μg/dL (1.14–1.75 μmol/L)
Ethanol, blood	<50 mg/dL (11 nmol/L)

Fibrinogen, plasma	150–350 mg/dL (1.5–3.5 g/L)
Folate, red cell	160–855 ng/mL (362–1937 nmol/L)
Folate, serum	2.5–20.0 ng/mL (5.7–45.3 nmol/L)
Glucose, plasma-fasting	70–105 mg/dL (3.9–5.8 mmol/L); 2 hours postprandial <140 mg/dL (7.8 mmol/L)
Homocysteine, plasma	Male: 4–16 μmol/L
	female: 3–14 μmol/L
Immunoglobulins	
IgG	640–1430 mg/dL (6.4–14.3 g/L)
IgG$_1$	280–1020 mg/dL (2.8–10.2 g/L)
IgG$_2$	60–790 ng/dL (0.6–7.9 g/L)
IgG$_3$	14–240 mg/dL (0.14–2.40 g/L)
IgG$_4$	11–330 ng/dL (0.11–3.30 g/L)
IgA	70–300 mg/dL (0.7–3.0 g/L)
IgM	20–140 mg/dL (0.2–1.4 g/L)
IgD	<8 mg/dL (0.1–0.4 mg/L)
IgE	0.01–0.04 mg/dL (0.1–0.4 mg/L)
Iron, serum	60–160 μg/dL (11–29 μmol/L)
Iron binding capacity, serum	250–460 μg/dL (45–82 μmol/L)
Lactate dehydrogenase, serum	60–100 U/L
Lactic acid, venous blood	6–16 mg/dL (0.67–1.80 mmol/L)
Lead, blood	<40 μg/dL (1.9 μmol/L)
Lipase, serum	<95 U/L
Magnesium, serum	1.5–2.4 mg/dL (0.62–0.99 mmol/L)
Manganese, serum	0.3–0.9 ng/mL (300–900 ng/L)
Methylmalonic acid, serum	150–370 nmol/L
Osmolality, plasma	275–295 mosm/kg H_2O
Phosphatase, acid, serum	0.5–5.5 U/L
Phosphatase, alkaline, serum	36–92 U/L
Phosphorus, inorganic, serum	3.0–4.5 mg/dL (0.97–1.45 mmol/L)
Potassium, serum	3.5–5.0 mEq/L (3.5–5.0 mmol/L)
Protein, serum	
Total	6.0–7.8 g/dL (60–78 g/L)
Albumin	3.5–5.5 g/dL (35–55 g/L)
Globulins	2.5–3.5 g/dL (25–35 g/L)
Alpha$_1$	0.2–0.4 g/dL (2–4 g/L)
Alpha$_2$	0.5–0.9 g/dL (5–9 g/L)
Beta	0.6–1.1 g/dL (6–11 g/L)
Gamma	0.7–1.7 g/dL (7–17 g/L)
Rheumatoid factor	<40 U/mL (<40 kU/L)
Sodium, serum	136–145 mEq/L (136–145 mmol/L)
Triglycerides	<250 mg/dL (2.82 mmol/L), desirable
Urea nitrogen, serum	8–20 mg/dL (2.9–7.1 mmol/L)
Uric acid, serum	2.5–8.0 mg/dL (0.15–0.47 mmol/L)
Vitamin B$_{12}$, serum	200–800 pg/mL (148–590 pmol/L)

Cerebrospinal Fluid

Cell count	0–5 cells/μL (0–5 $\times$ 10^6 cells/L)
Glucose	40–80 mg/dL (2.5–4.4 mmol/L)
	<40% of simultaneous plasma concentration is abnormal
Protein	15–60 mg/dL (150–600 mg/L)
Pressure (opening)	70–200 cm H_2O

Endocrine

Adrenocorticotropin (ACTH)	9–52 pg/mL (2–11 pmol/L)
Aldosterone, serum	
Supine	2–5 ng/dL (55–138 pmol/L)
Standing	7–20 ng/dL (194–554 pmol/L)
Aldosterone, urine	5–19 µg/24 h (13.9–52.6 nmol/24 h)
Catecholamines	Epinephrine (supine): <75 ng/L (410 pmol/L)
	norepinephrine (supine): 50–440 ng/L
	(296–2600 pmol/L)
Catecholamines, 24-hour, urine	<100 µg/m^2 per 24 h (591 nmol/m^2 per 24 h)
Cortisol	
Serum	8 A.M.: 8–20 µg/dL (221–552 nmol/L)
	5 P.M.: 3–13 µg/dL (83–359 nmol/L)
1 h after cosyntropin	>18 µg/dL (498 nmol/L); usually 8 µg/dL
	(221 nmol/L) or more above baseline
Overnight suppression test	<5 µg/dL (138 nmol/24 h)
Dehydroepiandrosterone sulfate, plasma	Male: 1.3–5.5 mg/mL (3.5–14.9 µmol/L)
	female: 0.6–3.3 mg/mL (1.6–8.9 µmol/L)
11-deoxycortisol, plasma	Basal: <5 µg/dL (145 nmol/L)
	after metyrapone: >7 µg/dL (203 nmol/L)
Estradiol, serum	Male: 10–30 pg/mL (37–110 pmol/L)
	female: day 1–10, 50–100 pmol/L;
	day 11–20, 50–200 pmol/L
	day 21–30, 70–150 pmol/L
Estriol, urine	>12 mg/24 h (42 µmol/day)
Follicle-stimulating hormone, serum	Male (adult): 5–15 mU/mL (5–15 U/L)
	female: follicular or luteal phase, 5–20 mU/mL
	(5–20 U/L)
	midcycle peak, 30–50 mU/mL (30–50 U/L)
	postmenopausal, >35 mU/mL (35 U/L)
Growth hormone, plasma	After oral glucose, <2 ng/mL (2 µg/L)
	response to provocative stimuli: >7 ng/mL
	(7 µg/L)
17-hydroxycorticosteroids, urine	Male: 3–10 mg/24 h (8.3–28 µmol/24 h)
(Porter-Silber)	female: 2–8 mg/24 h (5.5–22.1 µmol/24 h)
Insulin, serum (fasting)	5–20 mU/L (35–139 pmol/L)
17-ketosteroids, urine	Male: 8–22 mg/24 h (28–77 µmol/24 h)
	female: up to 15 µg/24 h (52 mmol/24 h)
Luteinizing hormone, serum	Male: 3–15 mU/mL (3–15 U/L)
	female: follicular or luteal phase, 5–22 mU/mL
	(3–15 U/L)
	midcycle peak, 30–250 mU/mL (30–250 U/L)
	postmenopausal, >30 mU/mL (30 U/L)
Metanephrine, urine	<1.2 mg/24 h (6.1 mmol/24 h)
Parathyroid hormone, serum	10–65 pg/mL (10–65 ng/L)
Progesterone	
Luteal	3–30 ng/mL (0.10–0.95 nmol/L)
Follicular	<1 ng/mL (0.03 nmol/L)
Prolactin, serum	Male: <15 ng/mL (15 mg/L)
	female: <20 ng/mL (20 mg/L)
Renin activity (angiotensin-I	Normal diet: supine, 0.3–1.9 ng/mL per h
radioimmunoassay), plasma	(0.3–1.9 µg/L per h) upright, 0.2–3.6 ng/mL
	per h (0.2–3.6 µg/L per h)
Sperm concentration	20–150 million/mL (20–50 × 10^9/L)
Sweat test for sodium and chloride	<60 mEq/L (60 mmol/L)

Testosterone, serum	Adult male: 300–1200 ng/dL (10–42 nmol/L)
	female: 20–75 ng/dL (0.7–2.6 nmol/L)
Thyroid function tests (normal ranges vary)	
Thyroid iodine (^{131}I) uptake	10%–30% of administered dose at 24 h
Thyroid-stimulating hormone (TSH)	0.5–5.0 μU/mL (0.5–5.0 mU/mL)
Thyroxine (T$_4$), serum	
Total	5–12 μg/dL (64–155 nmol/L)
Free	0.9–2.4 ng/dL (12–31 pmol/L)
Free T$_4$ index	4–11
Triiodothyronine, resin (T$_3$)	25%–35%
Triiodothyronine, serum (T$_3$)	70–195 ng/dL (1.1–3.0 nmol/L)
Vanillylmandelic acid, urine	<8 mg/24 h (40.4 μmol/24 h)
Vitamin D	
1,25-dihydroxy, serum	25–65 pg/mL (60–156 pmol/L)
25-hydroxy, serum	15–80 ng/mL (37–200 nmol/L)

Gastrointestinal

D-xylose absorption (after ingestion of 25 g of D-xylose)	Urine excretion: 5–8 g at 5 h (33–53 mmol)
	serum D-xylose: >20 mg/dL at 2 h (1.3 nmol/L)
Fecal urobilinogen	40–280 mg/24 h (68–473 μmol/24 h)
Gastric secretion	Basal secretion: male: 4.0 ± 0.2 mEq of HCl/h (4.0 ± 0.2 mmol/h)
	female: 2.1 ± 0.2 mEq of HCl/h (2.1 ± 0.2 mmol/h)
	peak acid secretion: male: 37.4 ± 0.8 mEq/h (37.4 ± 0.8 mmol/h)
	female: 24.9 ± 1.0 mEq/h (24.9 ± 1.0 mmol/h)
Gastrin, serum	0–180 pg/mL (0–180 ng/L)
Lactose tolerance test	Increase in plasma glucose: >15 mg/dL (0.83 mmol/L)
Lipase, ascitic fluid	<200 U/L
Secretin-cholecystokinin pancreatic function	>80 mEq/L (80 mmol/L) of HCO$_3$ in at least one specimen collected over 1 h
Stool fat	<5 g/day on a 100-g fat diet
Stool nitrogen	<2 g/day
Stool weight	<200 g/day

Hematology

Activated partial thromboplastin time	25–35 sec
Bleeding time	<10 min
Coagulation factors, plasma	
Factor I	150–350 mg/dL (1.5–3.5 g/L)
Factor II	60%–150% of normal
Factor V	60%–150% of normal
Factor VII	60%–150% of normal
Factor VIII	60%–150% of normal
Factor IX	60%–150% of normal
Factor X	60%–150% of normal
Factor XI	60%–150% of normal
Factor XII	60%–150% of normal
Erythrocyte count	4.2–5.9 million cells/μL (4.2–5.9 × 10^{12} cells/L)
Erythrocyte survival rate (^{51}Cr)	T$^1/_2$ = 28 days
Erythropoietin	<30 mU/mL (30 U/L)
D-dimer	<15–200 ng/mL (15–200 mg/L)
Ferritin, serum	15–200 ng/mL (15–200 mg/L)

Glucose-6-phosphate dehydrogenase, blood	5–15 U/g Hgb (0.32–0.97 mU/mol Hgb)
Haptoglobin, serum	50–150 mg/dL (500–1500 mg/L)
Hematocrit	Male: 41%–51%
	female: 36%–47%
Hemoglobin, blood	Male: 14–17 g/dL (140–170 g/L)
	female: 12–16 g/dL (120–160 g/L)
Hemoglobin, plasma	0.5–5.0 mg/dL (0.08–0.80 μmol/L)
Leukocyte alkaline phosphatase	15–40 mg of phosphorus liberated/ h per 10^{10} cells
	score $= 13$–130/100 polymorphonuclear neutrophils and band forms
Leukocyte count	Nonblacks: 4000–10,000/μL (4.0–10 $\times$ 10^9/L)
	blacks: 3500–10,000/μL (3.5–10 $\times$ 10^9/L)
Lymphocytes	
CD4$^+$ cell count	640–1175/μL (0.64–1.18 $\times$ 10^9/L)
CD4$^+$ cell count	335–875/μL (0.34–0.88 $\times$ 10^9/L)
CD4: CD8 ratio	1.0–4.0
Mean corpuscular hemoglobin (MCH)	28–32 pg
Mean corpuscular hemoglobin concentration (MCHC)	32–36 g/dL (320–360 g/L)
Mean corpuscular volume (MCV)	80–100 fL
Osmotic fragility of erythrocytes	Increased if hemolysis occurs in >0.5% NaCl, decreased if hemolysis is incomplete in 0.3% NaCl
Platelet count	150,000–350,000/μL (150–350 $\times$ 10^9/L)
Platelet life span (^{51}Cr)	8–12 days
Protein C activity, plasma	67%–131%
Protein C resistance	2.2–2.6
Protein S activity, plasma	82%–144%
Prothrombin time	11–13 sec
Reticulocyte count	0.5%–1.5% of erythrocytes
	absolute: 23,000–90,000 cells/μL (23–90 $\times$ 10^9/L)
Schilling test (oral administration of radioactive cobalamin-labeled vitamin B_{12})	8.5%–28.0% excreted in urine per 24–48 h
Sedimentation rate, erythrocyte (Westergren)	Male: 0–15 mm/h
	female: 0–20 mm/h
Volume, blood	
Plasma	Male: 25–44 mL/kg (0.025–0.044 L/kg) body weight
	female: 28–43 mL/kg (0.028–0.043 L/kg) body weight
Erythrocyte	Male: 25–35 mL/kg (0.025–0.044 L/kg) body weight
	female: 20–30 mL/kg (0.020–0.030 L/kg) body weight

Pulmonary

Forced expiratory volume in 1 second (FEV$_1$)	>80% predicted
Forced vital capacity (FVC)	>80% predicted
FEV$_1$/FVC	>75% (0.75)

Urine

Amino acids	200–400 mg/24 h (14–29 nmol/24 h)
Amylase	6.5–48.1 U/h

Calcium	100–300 mg/day (2.5–7.5 mmol/day) on unrestricted diet
Chloride	80–250 mEq/day (80–250 mmol/day) (varies with intake)
Copper	0–100 μg/24 h (0–1.6 μmol/day)
Coproporphyrin	50–250 μg/24 h (76–382 nmol/day)
Creatine	Male: 4–40 mg/24 h (30–305 mmol/24 h) female: 0–100 mg/24 h (0–763 mmol/h)
Creatinine	15–25 mg/kg per 24 h (133–221 mmol/ kg per 24 h)
Creatinine clearance	90–140 mL/min (0.09–0.14 L/min)
5-hydroxyindoleacetic acid (5-HIAA)	2–9 mg/24 h (10.4–46.8 μmol/day)
Osmolality	38–1400 mosm/kg H_2O
Phosphate, tubular resorption	79%–94% (0.79–0.94) of filtered load
Potassium	25–100 mEq/24 h (25–100 mmol/24 h) (varies with intake)
Protein	<100 mg/24 h
Sodium	100–260 mEq/24 h (100–260 mmol/24 h) (varies with intake)
Uric acid	250–270 mg/24 h (1.48–4.43 mmol/24 h) (varies with diet)
Urobilinogen	0.05–2.50 mg/24 h (0.08–4.22 μmol/24 h)

Reprinted with permission from MKSAP 12. American College of Physicians ©2002. All rights reserved.

1. A 44-year-old Hispanic man presents to your office for a routine yearly physical exam. His only concern is that his blood pressure was 153/88 at the local health fair 2 months ago. Past medical history is significant for moderate persistent asthma for which he takes daily fluticasone and albuterol as needed. He has been hospitalized twice in the last year for asthma exacerbations. On exam today his blood pressure is 155/90. The remainder of his cardiovascular and pulmonary exam is unremarkable. The best initial therapy for this patient's hypertension would be:

    A. Propranolol
    B. Diltiazem
    C. Hydrochlorothiazide
    D. Dietary modification and weight loss only
    E. Clonidine

2. A 29-year-old white woman presents with hypertension found during a pre-employment physical. She is otherwise asymptomatic. She has no prior medical history and takes no medications or herbal supplements. Blood pressure is 170/91. Funduscopic exam shows grade II hypertensive changes without hemorrhages. Cardiovascular and pulmonary exam is normal. Abdominal exam is remarkable for a bruit heard in the left upper quadrant. This patient's hypertension is most likely due to:

    A. Coronary artery disease
    B. Fibromuscular dysplasia of the renal artery
    C. Cushing's syndrome
    D. Benign essential hypertension
    E. Pheochromocytoma

The next two questions (items 3 and 4) correspond to the following vignette.

A 41-year-old white man presents with three weeks of progressive weight gain and pedal and periorbital edema. He has no prior medical history and takes no medications. Exam is notable for blood pressure of 151/92 with normal cardiovascular and pulmonary exam. 3+ Pedal edema is present. Lab studies are as follows: Creatinine 1.0 mg/dL; sodium 135 mEq/L; BUN 15 mg/dL; potassium 4.2 mEq/L; albumin 2.5 g/dL; urinalysis 4+ protein; no blood.

3. Which of the following additional studies should be ordered next to confirm the diagnosis?

    A. 24-hour urine protein
    B. Liver function tests
    C. Serum cholesterol
    D. Renal ultrasound
    E. Renal biopsy

4. What is the most common primary renal disease that causes this patient's syndrome in adult Americans?

    A. Minimal change disease
    B. Focal segmental glomerulosclerosis
    C. Membranoproliferative glomerulonephritis
    D. Membranous glomerulonephritis
    E. Amyloidosis

End of set

5. An 18-year-old man presents to your office with a complaint of hematuria. He also complains of an upper respiratory illness that began 2 days ago and consists of clear rhinorrhea, a nonproductive cough, and general myalgias. Blood pressure is 121/70 and he is afebrile. His nasal mucous membranes are mildly inflamed with clear rhinorrhea noted. His throat is mildly erythematous without tonsillar exudates. His heart is regular without murmurs, and his lungs are clear to auscultation. There are no skin rashes. A routine urinalysis shows 2+ blood and 1+ protein. Which of the following statements is true concerning this patient's disease process?

  A. Findings on renal biopsy would include mesangial proliferation and glomerular IgA deposits by immunofluorescence
  B. Serum IgA levels correlate with course of the disease
  C. The use of immunosuppressive treatment is well established
  D. 10% to 25% of patients have normal renal function 10 years after diagnosis
  E. The natural course of this disease is well known and predictable

6. A 34-year-old man presents with complaints of severe right flank pain that began 4 hours ago. The pain is sharp, severe, and radiates to the right groin. He denies fever and finds it difficult to urinate. On exam, he appears to be in distress secondary to pain. His pulse is 105 and his blood pressure is 148/90. He is afebrile. On physical exam, he has costovertebral angle tenderness over the right flank. The exam is otherwise normal. A urinalysis reveals a urine pH of 6.5, is positive for blood, and is negative for WBCs, leukocyte esterase, and nitrites. An abdominal plain film shows a small 3-mm radio-opaque density over the right flank. A stone is collected and sent for study. The composition of this patient's stone is most likely to be:

  A. Uric acid
  B. Struvite
  C. Cystine
  D. Calcium oxalate
  E. Calcium hydroxyapatite (HA)

7. A 76-year-old male nursing home patient with small cell lung cancer is brought into the ER for confusion worsening over the last 24 hours. He has no history of fever or recent medication changes. Vital signs reveal that the patient's blood pressure is 118/70, his pulse is 70, and he is afebrile. The exam is notable for a cachectic-appearing elderly man who is disoriented and unable to answer questions appropriately. Initial lab results are as follows: Sodium 113 mEq/L; glucose 95 mg/dL; calcium 9.0 mg/dL; magnesium 1.8 mEq/L. The patient begins to have a generalized tonic clonic seizure. Which of the following is the most appropriate initial management?

  A. Fluid restriction
  B. Infuse 3% hypertonic saline
  C. Start IV demeclocycline
  D. Give 1 ampule of dextrose 50 IV
  E. CT of the head

8. You are in the clinic and have ordered a urine dip on a patient with diabetes to evaluate for proteinuria. If this dip is negative for macroscopic protein, you plan on sending the urine for microalbumin levels. Which of the following statements regarding detecting proteinuria on urine dipstick testing is true?

A. A urine dipstick can detect protein in a concentrated urine specimen with the same accuracy as a dilute urine specimen

B. False-positive reactions may occur as a result of some antiseptics and other iodinated agents

C. Normal amounts of protein do not cause a positive reaction in a concentrated specimen

D. Highly acidic urine may cause false-positive reactions

E. Immunoglobulins or light chains in the urine can be reliably detected by urine dipstick

9. A 40-year-old man is admitted after a suicide attempt. He states that he drank a liquid substance found in his garage. He is unable to give more specific details. He is complaining of blurred vision. He is awake and alert with normal vital signs and normal physical exam. Labs are as follows: Glucose 90 mg/dL, sodium 140 mEq/L; potassium 4.9 mEq/L; chloride 95 mEq/L; bicarbonate 15 mEq/L; BUN 17 mg/dL; creatinine 1.3 mg/dL; osmolality 320; pH on arterial blood gas 7.28. No crystals are noted on urinalysis. What substance did this patient most likely ingest?

A. Mannitol
B. Ethylene glycol
C. Methanol
D. Gasoline
E. Isopropyl alcohol

10. A 65-year-old man with chronic renal insufficiency secondary to polycystic kidney disease presents with impaired mental status, nausea, and vomiting. He is disoriented to time and place on exam. Excoriated areas of skin and asterixis are also noted on physical exam. The patient's symptoms are most likely due to elevated:

A. Phosphorus
B. Potassium
C. BUN
D. Sodium
E. Bicarbonate

11. A 74-year-old man with congestive heart failure (CHF) presents with generalized weakness. He reports running out of his furosemide 4 days ago, but continuing all other medications including his angiotensin-converting enzyme (ACE) inhibitor, β-blocker, spironolactone, and potassium chloride supplement. Blood pressure is 125/85, and jugular venous distension is present. His cardiovascular exam is notable for a S_3 gallop, his lungs are clear to auscultation bilaterally, and he has 1+ pedal edema. An ECG is obtained (Figure 11). What is the most likely diagnosis?

A. Hypercalcemia
B. Acute myocardial infarction
C. Uncontrolled congestive heart failure
D. Hypokalemia
E. Hyperkalemia

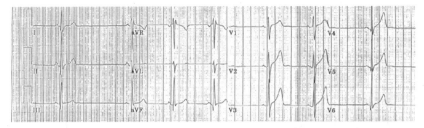

Figure 11 · Image courtesy of Dr. Brenda Shinar, Banner Good Samaritan Medical Center, Phoenix, Arizona

12. A 54-year-old man was admitted for abdominal pain, nausea, vomiting, and diarrhea for the past 2 days. He has been unable to tolerate any oral intake of food or water for the past 2 days. His blood pressure on admit was 90/50 with a pulse of 140, and his labs were significant for a creatinine of 2.0 mg/dL, which was up from his baseline of 1.0 mg/dL. Which of the following urine sediments is most suggestive of acute tubular necrosis?

A. Red blood cell casts
B. White blood cell casts
C. Muddy brown granular casts
D. Hyaline casts
E. Eosinophils

The response options for items 13 through 16 are the same. You will be required to select one answer for each item in the set.

A. pH 7.27, pCO_2 14 mmHg; bicarbonate 7 mEq/L; sodium 134 mEq/L; potassium 2.7 mEq/L; chloride 116 mEq/L
B. pH 7.0; pCO_2 72 mmHg; bicarbonate 15 mEq/L; sodium 138 mEq/L; potassium 5.7 mEq/L; chloride 90 mEq/L
C. pH 7.15; pCO_2 18 mmHg; bicarbonate 7 mEq/L; sodium 128 mEq/L; potassium 4.1 mEq/L; chloride 100 mEq/L
D. pH 7.52; pCO_2 23 mmHg; bicarbonate 20 mEq/L; sodium 135 mEq/L; potassium 4.2 mEq/L; chloride 108 mEq/L
E. E. pH 7.32; pCO_2 50 mmHg; bicarbonate 19 mEq/L; sodium 138 mEq/L; potassium 5.0 mEq/L; chloride 108 mEq/L

For each clinical scenario, select the most appropriate arterial blood gas and electrolyte values.

13. A 61-year-old man with diabetes presents with nausea, vomiting, and polyuria.

14. A 23-year-old woman presents with palpitations, chest pain, and an "impending sense of doom."

15. A 34-year-old woman presents with watery diarrhea for the last 3 days.

16. A 28-year-old man with history of asthma presents with tachypnea, wheezing, chest tightness, and severe shortness of breath.

End of set

17. A 55-year-old man is admitted to the hospital with hematemesis. He had no prior abdominal pain and has a significant history of alcohol abuse. You are concerned that the patient may have unrecognized severe liver disease and that his upper GI bleed may be due to esophageal varices. Which of the following is a physical exam finding in a patient with liver cirrhosis that may clue you to the correct etiology of his bleeding?

A. Buffalo hump
B. Palmar erythema
C. Palpable purpura
D. Proptosis
E. Acanthosis nigricans

18. An 18-year-old woman comes to your office with complaints of nausea, vomiting, fever, and right upper quadrant discomfort for the past 4 days. She noticed that the whites of her eyes began to turn yellow yesterday. She has no prior medical history, does not drink alcohol, smoke, or use drugs, and has never had sexual intercourse. She works in a day-care facility. On physical exam, her vital signs are the following: Blood pressure 105/70, heart rate 100, respiratory rate 14, and temperature 99.0°F (37.2°C). She has mild scleral icterus and her mucous membranes are dry. She has a normal cardiac and pulmonary exam, and abdominal exam reveals mild hepatomegaly with tenderness to moderate palpation in the right upper quadrant. There is no splenomegaly. Her laboratories reveal an AST of 1500 U/L, an ALT of 1700 U/L, and total bilirubin of 2.5 mg/dL. Her alkaline phosphase is normal at 80 U/L. You suspect a viral hepatitis. Which of the following is a risk factor for transmission of hepatitis A?

A. IV drug use
B. Tattoos
C. Blood transfusions
D. Work in a health care profession
E. Ingestion of fecally contaminated water

19. A 65-year-old white woman presents to your office with complaints of dysphagia for solids but not for liquids that seems to be getting worse for the past year. She has had to eliminate bread from her diet because of its tendency to get stuck, and to cut up her food in small pieces. She has also noted weight loss of 10 pounds in the last month. She has been taking an over-the-counter H2 blocker and other antacids for symptom relief of her heartburn, which she has had for over 10 years. Past medical history and family history are otherwise negative. The next step in this patient's care is:

A. 24-hour pH esophageal monitor
B. Endoscopy
C. Chest X-ray
D. CT scan of chest
E. Trial a proton pump inhibitor

20. A 46-year-old white woman presents to your office for routine checkup. Past medical history is significant for asthma diagnosed 2 years ago. She states she has an asthma attack two to three times per month, and the episodes usually occur at night. She has not noted any improvement with her current regimen of an albuterol metered dose inhaler. Further review of systems is otherwise negative with the exception of heartburn she has had for the past 3 years. Exam is essentially normal with no evidence of tachypnea or hypoxia. Lung fields are clear bilaterally without wheezes. There is no prolonged respiratory phase and no accessory muscle use. The next step in the treatment of this patient's bronchospasm is:

A. Add a long-acting β-agonist
B. Start an inhaled steroid
C. Add a leukotriene receptor antagonist
D. Trial a proton pump inhibitor
E. No change in therapy at this time

21. A 69-year-old white man presents to the ED with sudden onset of left lower quadrant pain, fever, nausea, and vomiting. He states the pain started 2 days ago. He denies any history of diarrhea, melena, or hematochezia and states that he has not had a bowel movement in 2 days, since the pain started. He says that his only medical problem is constipation. He denies any sick contacts. On exam he has a low-grade temperature of 100.3°F (37.9°C) with otherwise normal vital signs. Abdominal exam is significant for left lower quadrant tenderness to palpation with some fullness. Bowel sounds are hypoactive and there is no rebound. This patient most likely has:

A. Inflammatory bowel disease
B. Diverticulitis
C. Colon cancer
D. Diverticulosis
E. Appendicitis

22. A 76-year-old man comes to the ER with complaints of bright red blood per rectum (BRBPR). He says that it has occurred a couple of times in the past month, and he has noticed some blood surrounding the stool or on the toilet paper. This morning there appeared to be quite a bit of blood in the toilet and the patient said he got a little light-headed. He denies abdominal pain, fever, weight loss, or bleeding at any other site. On physical exam, he is not orthostatic. His abdominal exam is normal, and his rectal exam reveals a small amount of bright red blood. What is the most common cause of lower GI bleeding and therefore his most likely diagnosis?

A. Diverticulosis
B. Hemorrhoids
C. Infectious diarrhea
D. Inflammatory bowel disease
E. Upper GI bleed

23. A 35-year-old white man presents with a 2- to 3-week history of odynophagia. Past medical history is significant for AIDS diagnosed 5 years ago. The patient notes pain with swallowing of both liquids and solids. He denies any sensation of food getting stuck. He has lost approximately 5 pounds secondary to inability to eat. The most likely cause of this person's odynophagia is:

    A. Gastroesophageal reflux disease (GERD)
    B. Achalasia
    C. Barrett's esophagus
    D. Infectious esophagitis
    E. Diffuse esophageal spasms

24. An 82-year-old woman comes to your clinic with complaints of fatigue and shortness of breath for the past couple of months. She has also noticed that she is not as hungry as usual and when she does eat, she gets full quickly. She denies abdominal pain, chest pain, or cough. She has lost approximately 15 pounds over the past 6 months without intention, but she attributes it to not eating as much. On physical exam, she is thin and in no acute distress. She has normal vital signs. Her exam is unremarkable, including her abdominal exam, although her rectal exam reveals brown, guaiac-positive stool. Her laboratories reveal a microcytic, microchromic anemia with a hemoglobin of 9.2. She is referred for upper and lower endoscopy, and the upper endoscopy reveals a 4-cm ulcerated mass in the antrum of the stomach. Which of the following is an independent risk factor for gastric adenocarcinoma?

    A. Alcohol abuse
    B. Nonsteroidal anti-inflammatory drug (NSAID)-induced ulcers
    C. Tobacco abuse
    D. Long-standing GERD
    E. *Helicobacter pylori*

25. A 45-year-old obese white woman presents with severe epigastric pain radiating to her back. She states the symptoms started yesterday and are also associated with vomiting. She denies any fever or chills. She also denies any change in bowel habits. On review of systems she states that intermittently she has right-sided abdominal pain after eating out at her favorite Mexican restaurant. She denies any history of alcohol abuse. Physical exam is essentially within normal limits with the exception of her abdomen, which is tender to palpation in the epigastric region. There is no rebound or hepatosplenomegaly. Bowel sounds are normoactive. You order basic labs that reveal normal liver function tests; however, the patient does have an elevated amylase and lipase. The most likely cause of her pancreatitis is:

    A. Gallstones
    B. Alcohol use
    C. Trauma
    D. Drugs
    E. Tobacco use

26. An 18-year-old white man presents with 2 to 3 days of diarrhea. He denies any recent travel but recently dined at a new restaurant with his family. No other sick contacts are noted. He states the diarrhea is blood-tinged and loose in nature. He complains of crampy abdominal pain. On physical exam the patient is afebrile, heart rate is 96, respiratory rate is 18, and blood pressure is 120/72. In general he is alert, pale appearing, and in no acute distress. HEENT exam is significant for pale conjunctivae. Chest is clear, and cardiovascular exam reveals a regular rate and rhythm with a II/VI systolic ejection murmur at the left sternal border. Abdomen is soft with diffuse tenderness and skin exam reveals multiple petechiae on his lower extremities. Labs are as follows: WBCs 15,000/µl; hemoglobin 8.0 g/dL; hematocrit 23.0; platelets 40,000; BUN 100; creatinine 7.8. The infectious organism that would best explain the patient's syndrome is:

A. *Cryptosporidium*
B. *Giardia*
C. Rotavirus
D. *E. coli* O157:H7
E. *Vibrio cholerae*

27. A 24-year-old white woman presents to your office with intermittent, cramping abdominal pain with alternating diarrhea, constipation, and bloating. These symptoms have occurred for the past 3 years and she notes that the symptoms get worse when she is stressed. She denies any family history of colon problems. You suspect irritable bowel syndrome. Which of the following is included in the Rome Diagnostic Criteria for irritable bowel syndrome?

A. Abdominal pain causing nighttime awakening
B. Passage of mucus
C. Steatorrhea
D. Bloody stool
E. Weight loss

28. A 65-year-old white man presents to your ED with sudden-onset severe periumbilical pain. He denies any fevers, diarrhea, or constipation. Past medical history is significant for atrial fibrillation for which he is on aspirin. On physical exam patient is in severe, distressing pain. He is afebrile, with an irregular tachycardia at 160, and a blood pressure of 120/90. In general he is ill appearing and his abdominal exam is significant for hypoactive bowel sounds, with mild tenderness to palpation. His rectal exam reveals brown, guaiac-positive stool. The most likely cause of this man's abdominal pain is:

A. Diffuse atherosclerosis
B. Arterial embolism
C. Venous thrombosis
D. Ischemic colitis
E. Small bowel obstruction

29. A 68 year-old white woman presents with a six-month history of weight loss and hematochezia. She states her last colonoscopy was approximately 5 years ago and a hyperplastic polyp was seen at that time. You refer her for colonoscopy and a 4-cm mass is seen in the proximal sigmoid colon. The pathology of the biopsy specimens is confirmed as adenocarcinoma of the colon. A CT scan of the chest, abdomen, and pelvis is performed and shows no evidence of metastatic disease. The next step for this patient includes:

 A. Surveillance colonoscopy every 6 months
 B. Surgery for staging and excision
 C. Chemotherapy
 D. Radiation therapy
 E. MRI of the brain to rule out metastases

30. A 40-year-old white woman comes to your office for a preventative care visit. In general she is doing well without any complaints. She takes no medications. She is active, playing tennis three times weekly. She is trying to cut down on red meats, but finds this difficult when cooking for her husband. She does not smoke, but does enjoy 3 to 4 glasses of wine weekly. Her father was diagnosed with colon cancer at age 60. What is (or would have been) the appropriate colon cancer screening recommendations for her?

 A. Colonoscopy every 3 to 5 years, starting at age 30
 B. Fecal occult blood testing (FOBT) annually, sigmoidoscopy every 3 to 5 years, or colonoscopy every 10 years, starting at age 40
 C. FOBT and sigmoidoscopy every 3 to 5 years, colonoscopy every 10 years, starting at age 50
 D. Sigmoidoscopy every 1 to 2 years, starting at age 12
 E. FOBT every year, no need for sigmoidoscopy or colonoscopy

31. A 30-year-old woman comes to your office with complaints of a skin rash on her lower legs that she has noticed for the past three weeks while shaving. She has also noted a few nosebleeds that have occurred spontaneously and have been difficult to stop, over the same time period. She has no other complaints of fever or fatigue. On physical exam, her vital signs are normal. She has petechiae on her soft palate and conjunctivae are pink. Her heart, lungs, and abdominal exams are normal. Her lower extremities reveal a nonblanching petechial rash. You suspect idiopathic thrombocytopenic purpura (ITP). Which of the follow statements is true regarding ITP?

 A. Peak age of occurrence is in the third decade
 B. First line therapy is splenectomy
 C. IV immunoglobulin (IVIG) has been shown to increase platelet counts in 60% to 70% of patients
 D. It is caused by a membrane defect of the platelets
 E. Persistence of thrombocytopenia for more than 3 months is considered chronic autoimmune thrombocytopenia

The response options for items 32 through 42 are the same. You will be required to select one answer for each item in the set.

A. HIV infection
B. Cryoglobulinemia
C. Sarcoidosis
D. Diabetes mellitus
E. Hepatitis B
F. Hepatitis C
G. Herpes simplex virus
H. *Pseudomonas aeruginosa*
I. Celiac sprue
J. Systemic lupus erythematosus (SLE)
K. Reiter's syndrome
L. Inflammatory bowel disease
M. Syphilis
N. Lyme disease

For each skin lesion, select the systemic disorder with which it is associated.

32. Pyoderma gangrenosum

33. Acanthosis nigricans

34. Erythema nodosum

35. Erythema multiforme

36. Seborrheic dermatitis

37. Ecthyma gangrenosum

38. Erythema migrans

39. Condyloma lata

40. Dermatitis herpetiformis

41. Keratoderma blennorrhagicum

42. Porphyria cutanea tarda

End of set

43. A 70-year-old man with no significant past medical history is brought to your office by his wife for complaints of "forgetfulness." His wife tells you that for the past year she has noticed a decline in his short-term memory and cognitive abilities. He has been unable to balance the checkbook as he used to do and is easily frustrated and often irritable, which is not his usual personality. His occupation was real estate sales until he retired approximately 5 years ago. On physical exam, his blood pressure is 150/85, heart rate is 80, and respiratory rate is 14. He is afebrile. He scores a 24/30 on Mini-Mental State exam (MMSE). His neurologic exam reveals a pleasant affect, and he is alert and oriented to person, place, and time. His cranial nerves are intact, and there are no tremors or cogwheel rigidity. His gait is slow, slightly broad based, and he seems to have difficulty coordinating his foot movements. Reflexes are within normal limits, and the rest of the physical exam is within normal limits. Laboratories reveal a normal TSH, B_{12} level, BUN, creatinine, AST, ALT, bilirubin, and CBC. Which of the following diagnoses is most likely, and what test is the best test to evaluate for it?

    A. Normal pressure hydrocephalus (NPH); CT scan of the brain
    B. Multi-infarct dementia; MRI of the brain
    C. Diffuse Lewy-body disease; brain biopsy
    D. Pick's disease; CT of the brain
    E. Supranuclear palsy; MRI of the brain

44. A 63-year-old man is admitted to the hospital with fever, malaise, and abdominal pain. His past medical history is significant for hyperlipidemia for which he takes pravastatin. He was in his usual state of health until several months ago when he noted unintentional, gradual weight loss, fatigue, and night sweats. These symptoms began to worsen 1 week before admission. He developed abdominal pain the day of admission that prompted him to seek medical attention. On evaluation of the patient you find the following: Temperature 101.1°F (38.4°C); pulse 94; respirations 16; blood pressure 138/72. Head and neck examination reveals several conjunctival petechiae. His heart examination reveals a III/VI systolic murmur at the right upper sternal border. The patient does not recall being told of a heart murmur in the past. Lung examination is normal. Extremity examination reveals erythematous, macular lesions on several of his fingers that are not tender. Abdominal examination reveals tenderness in the left upper quadrant but normal bowel sounds and no rebound or guarding. You suspect infective endocarditis. You order blood cultures and a transthoracic echocardiogram. Blood cultures are positive for *Streptococcus bovis* in all bottles. Echocardiogram reveals a 4-mm vegetation on the aortic valve. What is the next step in the care of this patient?

    A. Transesophageal echocardiogram
    B. Computed tomography of the abdomen and pelvis
    C. Colonoscopy
    D. Evaluation by a cardiothoracic surgeon
    E. Skin biopsy of lesions on fingers

45. A 45-year-old woman presents to the ED with a 2-day history of left lower extremity pain and swelling and pleuritic chest pain and shortness of breath. She has no past medical history. Oral contraceptives are her only medication. She smokes one pack of cigarettes per day. You suspect a deep venous thrombosis with pulmonary embolism and order a ventilation perfusion scan. While waiting for the scan to be done you receive her arterial blood gas results and they show the following: paO_2 58 mmHg; $paCO_2$ 30 mmHg; pH 7.48 on room air. What is her alveolar-arterial (A-a) oxygen gradient?

A. 68
B. 48
C. There is not enough information to calculate the A-a gradient
D. 130
E. 55

46. A 62-year-old woman presents to the ED with complaints of sudden onset of dizziness and shortness of breath. Her past medical history is significant for hypertension and diabetes mellitus. On exam, she is afebrile and has a blood pressure of 74/42 with a heart rate of 138. On exam, her lungs have bibasilar crackles and her heart rate is irregularly irregular with no murmurs noted. You obtain an electrocardiogram (Figure 46). The most important initial step in her management is:

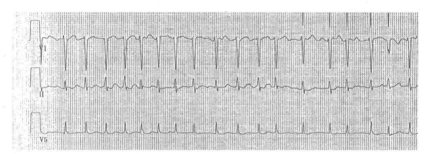

Figure 46 • Image courtesy of Dr. Brenda Shinar, Banner Good Samaritan Medical Center, Phoenix, Arizona

A. Initiation of warfarin therapy
B. Rate control with IV calcium-channel blockers
C. Initiation of aspirin therapy
D. Cardioversion of her rhythm with amiodarone
E. Synchronized electrical cardioversion

47. A 21-year-old previously healthy man collapses while playing basketball with his friends. Paramedics are called, and he is found to be in pulseless ventricular tachycardia and is defibrillated with success. He is intubated and transferred to the ED where he is found to have a blood pressure of 118/80 with a heart rate of 94. His exam reveals a tall, thin man with a harsh midsystolic murmur over the middle upper right sternal area. An ECG reveals evidence for mild left ventricular hypertrophy (LVH) with no evidence of ischemia. A chest X-ray is normal. His mother arrives and tells you that he had an older sibling who suffered sudden cardiac death. What is the most likely cause of his clinical picture?

A. Ventricular septal defect (VSD)
B. Pulmonary embolus
C. Tension pneumothorax
D. Hypertrophic obstructive cardiomyopathy (HCM)
E. Dissecting aortic aneurysm

48. A 19-year-old woman presents to your office with complaints of progressive dyspnea on exertion and fatigue. Her symptoms started approximately 3 weeks earlier. On examination, you find that she has a blood pressure of 176/98 measured in her right arm. Upon auscultation, you notice a midsystolic murmur that is also heard in her upper back area. A repeat blood pressure measurement in her left arm confirms your earlier findings. You obtain an ECG that shows criteria for LVH. A chest X-ray obtained in the office shows absence of the aortic notch with notching of the ribs. What is the likely diagnosis?

A. Atrial septal defect (ASD)
B. Coarctation of the aorta
C. Aortic stenosis (AS)
D. Patent ductus arteriosus (PDA)
E. HCM

49. You have volunteered to do sports physicals on the athletes at your son's high school to clear them for participation in the competitive events. One of the varsity basketball players is a 16-year-old man without any significant past medical history. You hear a 2/6 systolic murmur in the right upper sternal border. The patient thinks that he was told that he had a heart murmur, but he is unsure. You are worried that there may be a contraindication to him playing basketball. You must have the patient do several maneuvers and be able to interpret them to know the etiology of his murmur. The Valsalva maneuver will make which of the following murmurs louder?

A. HCM
B. AS
C. Aortic insufficiency (AI)
D. Mitral stenosis
E. Tricuspid stenosis

50. A 65-year-old woman with a history of diabetes and hypertension developed chest pain while shoveling her snowy front walk in the early morning. The pain is 8/10 in severity with a "pressure-like" quality and is radiating a little to the jaw. It has persisted for 2 hours. The patient finally called 911 and paramedics brought her to the ER. An ECG reveals normal sinus rhythm without any acute ST-T wave changes. You appropriately treat the patient empirically for an acute coronary syndrome, and she is admitted to telemetry to "rule out" a myocardial infarction. In which order, from first to last, would you expect the following markers to peak after an acute myocardial infarction?

A. Troponin-I, LDH, myoglobin, CPK-MB
B. Troponin-I, myoglobin, CPK-MB, LDH
C. Myoglobin, CPK-MB, troponin-I, LDH
D. Myoglobin, troponin-I, CPK-MB, LDH
E. Myoglobin, LDH, troponin-I, CPK-MB

Answers and Explanations

ONE

Answer Key

1.	C	18.	E	35.	G
2.	B	19.	B	36.	A
3.	A	20.	D	37.	H
4.	D	21.	B	38.	N
5.	A	22.	A	39.	M
6.	D	23.	D	40.	I
7.	B	24.	E	41.	K
8.	B	25.	A	42.	F
9.	C	26.	D	43.	A
10.	C	27.	B	44.	C
11.	E	28.	B	45.	E
12.	C	29.	B	46.	E
13.	C	30.	B	47.	D
14.	D	31.	C	48.	B
15.	A	32.	L	49.	A
16.	E	33.	D	50.	C
17.	B	34.	C		

1. **C.** This patient has hypertension confirmed by two measurements, warranting pharmacologic therapy. First-line medications for hypertension include β-blockers and thiazide diuretics. With this patient's history of asthma, the diuretic would be a better choice for first-line therapy.

A. A β-blocker, especially a nonselective β-blocker, would be contraindicated in this patient with asthma.

B. Calcium channel blockers are not first-line therapy for hypertension. Long-acting calcium channel blockers may be added to the medication regimen if first-line therapy does not control the blood pressure or if the patient is unable to tolerate first-line medications.

D. According to the JNC VII guidelines, drug therapy is indicated for stage I hypertension. Stage I hypertension is defined as a systolic blood pressure of 140–159 or diastolic blood pressure of 90–99. Lifestyle modifications should also be encouraged, but not used alone.

E. A centrally acting adrenergic drug is not considered first-line therapy for hypertension.

2. **B.** This patient has features suggestive of a secondary cause for her hypertension including age of onset less than 30, abrupt onset, findings on funduscopic exam, and an abdominal bruit. The abdominal bruit suggests a narrowing of the renal artery. The most common cause of hypertension secondary to renal artery stenosis in young women is fibromuscular dysplasia of the renal artery. (The most common cause of renal artery stenosis in an older population is atherosclerotic disease.)

A. Hypertension is a cause of coronary artery disease, not the reverse.

C. Although Cushing's syndrome is a cause of secondary hypertension, there are no findings on physical exam such as abdominal striae, buffalo hump, or moon facies to suggest Cushing's syndrome as a cause of this patient's hypertension.

D. This patient has features suggestive of a secondary cause for her hypertension. Further workup should be done to exclude secondary causes of hypertension before a diagnosis of essential hypertension is made.

E. There are no other features, including headaches, palpitations, or anxiety, to suggest a pheochromocytoma.

3. **A.** This patient has significant proteinuria on urinalysis and other findings consistent with nephrotic syndrome. Nephrotic syndrome is defined as urinary protein concentration of greater than 3.0 to 3.5 g over 24 hours. Additional features include hypoalbuminemia, edema, and hyperlipidemia.

B. Although abnormal liver function can cause hypoalbuminemia, the urinalysis suggests a renal cause for this patient's low albumin.

C. Elevated cholesterol is one of the findings in nephrotic syndrome. In nephrotic syndrome, proteinuria leads to hypoalbuminemia and decreased plasma oncotic pressure. This drop in oncotic pressure then stimulates liver lipoprotein synthesis, resulting in hyperlipidemia. However, there are other causes of elevated cholesterol, and serum cholesterol alone cannot confirm the diagnosis of nephrotic syndrome.

D. Imaging will not aid in establishing the diagnosis.

E. Biopsy can be used to establish the etiology of the nephrotic syndrome, but is not the initial study of choice to confirm the diagnosis.

4. | **D.** Membranous glomerulonephritis accounts for 30% to 40% of adult nephrotic syndrome. Biopsy is characterized by thickened glomerular capillary loops. Appropriate renal function is retained at 10 years in 70% of patients with this diagnosis.

A. Minimal change disease is the most common cause of nephrotic syndrome in children. Biopsy shows no abnormalities on light microscopy, but effacement of foot processes along capillary loops can be seen on electron microscopy.

B. Focal segmental glomerulosclerosis is the most common cause of nephrotic syndrome in black adults. Renal biopsy shows glomerulosclerosis. Many patients with this diagnosis progress to renal failure.

C. Membranoproliferative glomerulonephritis is a less common cause of nephrotic syndrome. Biopsy will show proliferation of the mesangial cells.

E. Amyloidosis causes renal disease by deposition of immunoglobulin light chains in the kidneys. This can lead to nephrotic syndrome and renal failure. Congo red stain can be used on renal biopsy to show amyloid deposition. Amyloidosis is a *secondary* cause of renal disease leading to nephrotic syndrome, and not a *primary* renal disorder. The most common secondary cause of nephrotic syndrome is diabetes mellitus.

5. | **A.** This patient has history and findings consistent with IgA nephropathy. IgA nephropathy can present as asymptomatic hematuria with or without proteinuria *immediately* after, or concomitant with, an upper respiratory tract infection. (This helps distinguish it from poststreptococcal glomerulonephritis that usually occurs a couple of weeks *after* the pharyngitis.) IgA nephropathy also may present in young adults as hematuria that follows vigorous exercise. Biopsy is usually not necessary. However, if a biopsy were to be done, findings would be consistent with those listed in answer choice A.

B. Serum IgA levels do not correlate with the progression of disease.

C. The role of immunosuppressive treatment in IgA nephropathy is not well defined, but is currently under investigation.

D. It is estimated that 80% of patients have normal renal function 10 years after diagnosis.

E. The course of IgA nephropathy is not constant and can include progression to renal failure, slow decline of renal function over years, or little to no change in renal function.

6. **D.** This patient has a typical presentation of nephrolithiasis. 75% of all kidney stones are composed of calcium oxalate or calcium phosphate. Calcium oxalate stones are radio-opaque and are more common in males. Other risk factors for calcium oxalate stones include hypercalciuria, low urine output, hyperuricosuria, hyperoxaluria, and low urine citrate concentrations. In some cases, a cause of the stone is not known.

A. Uric acid stones occur because of the presence of elevated uric acid in the urine. Findings with uric acid stones include an acidic urine pH and radiolucent stone. Uric acid stones account for approximately 5% to 10% of stones in the United States.

B. Struvite stones occur with infections of the urinary tract due to urease-producing bacteria (such as *Proteus* species). This patient does not have indices on the urinalysis that would suggest an infection. Urine pH is usually alkaline. Stones are radio-opaque and can progress to form staghorn calculus. Struvite stones are responsible for 10% to 15% of stones and occur more commonly in women.

C. Cystine stones occur rarely, causing 1% of all kidney stones. It is unlikely that the patient has this type of stone. They occur in patients with defects in renal tubular absorption of cystine, ornithine, arginine, or lysine, and they usually present earlier in life.

E. Calcium HA is the primary mineral of bone and teeth. Abnormal deposition of calcium HA is seen in areas of tissue damage (large muscle hematomas) or in joints of elderly patients. It usually causes a destructive arthropathy, especially in the knees, shoulders, hips, and fingers. Diagnosis is made by electron microscopy of synovial fluid or tissue that identifies the small, nonbirefringent crystals. There is not an association with nephrolithiasis.

7. **B.** This patient has symptomatic hyponatremia. Symptoms of hyponatremia include nausea, vomiting, irritability, mental confusion, and seizures. Hypertonic saline should be given to increase the serum sodium above 120 mEq/L or until asymptomatic. The total mEq of sodium required to increase plasma sodium concentration can be calculated by using the following formula.

$$Sodium\ required\ (mEq) = total\ body\ water\ (L) \times desired\ change\ in\ sodium\ (mEq/L)$$

Total body water averages 60% of body weight. (To calculate total body water, multiply this patients' weight in kilograms by 0.6.) If this patients weighs 70 kg, to raise the serum sodium from 113 to 120 mEq/L (a change of 7 meq) the mEq sodium required = 70(0.6) × 7, or 294 mEq of sodium. Hypertonic (3%) saline contains 513 mEq of sodium per liter. This patient only requires 294 mEq of sodium to increase his serum sodium to 120 mEq/L. To calculate how much hypertonic saline, in liters, he requires, divide 294 mEq by 513 mEq/liter. Thus, approximately 570 mL of hypertonic saline can be infused to correct this patient's sodium. In symptomatic patients, sodium should be corrected at a rate of 1.5 to 2 mEq/hour for the first 3 to 4 hours or until the patient is asymptomatic.

A. Fluid restriction would be appropriate management for an asymptomatic patient with SIADH. However, this patient is symptomatic and requires immediate intervention to raise his serum sodium.

C. Demeclocycline can be used in the treatment of SIADH refractory to fluid restriction. This drug acts on the collecting tubule by decreasing the response to antidiuretic hormone, causing increased free water excretion.

D. This patient's glucose level is normal. Therefore, the seizure is not secondary to hypoglycemia and giving glucose is of no benefit.

E. A CT of the head would not be indicated at this time because the low sodium appears to be the cause of the patient's seizure.

8. | **B.** Some antiseptic washes that contain iodine can cause a false-positive reaction for protein on urine dip. Additionally, false positives can occur when iodinated radiocontrast agents have been given in the last 24 hours.

A. Highly concentrated urine can cause a false-positive reaction for protein on urine dip. Highly dilute urine will underestimate the amount of proteinuria.

C. Urine dip can detect protein as low as 15 mg/dL. If the urine is concentrated, urine dip may be positive with normal levels of protein in the urine.

D. Highly alkaline urine can cause false-positive reactions.

E. Urine dipstick detects urine albumin. It may not react with immunoglobulins or light chains in the urine. These must be detected by use of sulfosalicylic acid, which will cause the urine to become turbid and cloudy if protein is present. An alternative that identifies other proteins in the urine besides albumin is urine protein electrophoresis (UPEP).

9. | **C.** Mannitol, ethylene glycol, methanol, and isopropyl alcohol all produce a serum osmolal gap. Methanol and ethylene glycol also produce an anion gap metabolic acidosis. The absence of urine crystals and complaint of blurred vision point to methanol as the substance that was ingested. Anion gap is calculated by the following equation.

$$Anion\ gap = [sodium\ (mEq/L)] - ([chloride\ (mEq/L)] + [bicarbonate\ (mEq/L)])$$

The anion gap in this patient is 30. Osmolality can be calculated by the following equation.

$$Plasma\ Osm\ (mOsm/kg) = 2 \times [Na + (mOsm/L)] + [BUN\ (mg/dL)/2.8] + [glucose\ (mg/dL)/18]$$

Osmolal gap is equal to the measured serum osmolality minus the calculated osmolality. This patient's osmolal gap = 320 mOsm/kg (measured) − 292 mOsm/kg (calculated), which equals 38 mOsm/kg. Any value over 10 is abnormal.

A. Mannitol can produce an osmolal gap, but does not produce an anion gap metabolic acidosis.

B. Ethylene glycol ingestion does produce an anion gap acidosis with osmolal gap. However, calcium oxalate crystals can be found on urinalysis with ethylene glycol ingestion, and patients do not typically complain of visual changes. Other manifestations include change in mental status and renal failure.

D. Gasoline is usually inhaled if used as a substance of abuse. It may produce nausea, vomiting, and cardiovascular and respiratory effects. The associated metabolic disturbances are not well documented.

E. Isopropyl alcohol produces an osmolal gap, but without an anion gap metabolic acidosis.

10.
C. This patient is uremic and in symptomatic renal failure. Symptoms of uremia include anorexia, nausea, emesis, an unpleasant "metallic" taste in the mouth (known as "dysgeusia"), asterixis, encephalopathy, seizures, pruritus, sleepiness, and impaired mental status. Uremic frost may be seen on the skin secondary to urea crystallization of sweat. Note that *uremia* is different from *azotemia*. Azotemia is an elevation of the BUN alone. Uremia is an elevation of the BUN along with the mentioned symptoms of nausea, pruritus, etc.

A. Hyperphosphatemia does not present with these symptoms. It is usually associated with an underlying disease process such as renal failure.

B. Hyperkalemia presents with neuromuscular weakness, cardiac arrhythmias, and tall peaked T waves on ECG.

D. Hypernatremia presents with mental status changes that can progress to seizures, coma, and death. Pruritus and asterixis are not present.

E. Elevated bicarbonate does not produce the symptoms noted in this patient.

11.
E. This patient has history and ECG findings consistent with hyperkalemia. Symptoms include muscles weakness and fatigue. More severe hyperkalemia can lead to cardiac manifestations. ECG will show peaked T waves that progress to a widened QRS, and ventricular fibrillation. Each of the medicines that he was using for heart failure can predispose to hyperkalemia, with the exception of the furosemide, which he stopped.

A. Symptoms of hypercalcemia include abdominal pain, constipation, nausea, and muscle weakness. A shortened QT interval can be found on ECG.

B. This patient does not complain of chest pain, shortness of breath, or diaphoresis. The electrocardiograph does not show any ST elevation or depression that would suggest cardiac ischemia.

C. Symptoms of uncontrolled CHF include peripheral edema and shortness of breath. Physical exam findings would include an elevated jugular venous pressure, S_3 gallop, crackles on pulmonary exam, and peripheral edema. ECG may show evidence of left ventricular hypertrophy. This patient has findings consistent with CHF, but appears to be stable and without evidence of acute worsening.

D. Symptoms of hypokalemia can include muscle cramps, slow bowel motility, and respiratory muscle paralysis. On ECG, T waves can be flat or inverted, and U waves may be present. Severe hypokalemia can lead to ventricular arrhythmias.

12. C. Muddy brown granular casts are most suggestive of acute tubular necrosis. These casts are made of renal tubular cells that have suffered an acute injury, formed casts, and have now become part of the urine sediment. Muddy brown casts do not change the color of the urine but are seen on microscopy. Grossly muddy-brown urine may be seen in rhabdomyolysis.

A. Red cell casts indicate glomerulonephritis.

B. White blood cell casts suggest acute interstitial nephritis or pyelonephritis.

D. Hyaline casts are nonspecific and not indicative of renal disease. These casts can be seen in concentrated urine, after exercise, or during diuretic therapy.

E. Urine eosinophils are seen in acute interstitial nephritis, although they are only 70% sensitive for this disorder and 83% specific. Other causes of eosinophiluria are renal atheroembolic disease, rapidly progressive glomerulonephritis, and acute prostatitis.

13. C. This patient is presenting with diabetic ketoacidosis. The labs show an elevated anion gap metabolic acidosis with appropriate respiratory compensation. Anion gap is calculated by the following equation.

$$Anion\ gap = [sodium(mEq/L)] - ([chloride\ (mEq/L)] + [bicarbonate\ (mEq/L)])$$

Normal anion gap is 8 to 12. Our patient's anion gap is 21. Respiratory compensation for metabolic acidosis can be calculated by using Winter's formula:

$$Change\ in\ pCO_2 = 1.5 \times [bicarbonate\ (mEq/L)] + 8(+/- 2)$$

Our patient's predicted pCO_2 equals $1.5 \times 7 + 8 = 18.5$. Our patient has appropriate compensation.

14. D. This patient is having an anxiety attack, causing her to hyperventilate. The blood gas reveals an acute respiratory alkalosis and no other electrolyte abnormalities.

15. A. This patient has metabolic acidosis without an elevated anion gap. This can be secondary to GI bicarbonate losses with diarrhea, such as in this patient. It can also be secondary to renal bicarbonate losses such as in a renal tubular acidosis.

16. E. This patient has an acute respiratory acidosis secondary to status asthmaticus. There are no other electrolyte abnormalities and no metabolic compensation because this is acute.

B. This blood gas and electrolyte panel reflects a patient with a combined anion-gap metabolic acidosis and a respiratory acidosis.

17. **B.** Palmar erythema and spider telangiectasias are found in patients with liver disease due to the hyperestrogenic state. This also accounts for the testicular atrophy in men and loss of axillary hair. Findings of portal hypertension in liver disease include ascites, esophageal varices, caput medusa, and hemorrhoids (nonspecific).

A. A buffalo hump is commonly seen on physical exam in a patient with cortisol excess or Cushing's syndrome. Other clinical manifestations include obesity, striae, and easy bruising.

C. Palpable purpura are characteristic of vasculitic processes including Henoch-Schönlein purpura and hypersensitivity vasculitis.

D. Proptosis is a physical exam finding seen with thyroid hormone excess and patients with Graves' disease.

E. Acanthosis nigricans is a clinical exam finding seen with insulin resistance or diabetes mellitus type II. Typically it is a velvety darkening of the skin at the nape of the neck and in the axilla.

18. **E.** Hepatitis A is transmitted by fecal-oral route through ingestion of fecally contaminated water or foodstuffs. Those at risk include travelers, children and workers at day care, and military personnel.

A, B, C, D. IV drug use, the presence of a tattoo, history of blood transfusions, and work in the health care profession are all risk factors for hepatitis B and hepatitis C transmission.

19. **B.** This patient may have an esophageal cancer given the history of dysphagia, weight loss, and history of heartburn. Endoscopy is the first step in a patient with dysphagia and other warning symptoms for cancer. Biopsy can be performed at the time of endoscopy to confirm diagnosis.

A. Twenty-four hour pH esophageal monitoring is the gold standard test for the diagnosis of gastroesophageal reflux disease; however, it would not be the appropriate next step in this patient because of the concern for cancer.

C. Chest X-ray may help if there is a large mass lesion in the patient's chest, but it would not provide direct visualization of tissue for diagnosis.

D. Similar to chest X-ray, CT scan of the chest would help determine if there was a mass lesion causing compression and extraesophageal dysphagia. CT would help delineate between anatomic structures better than plain films, but CT is not the gold standard in the evaluation of dysphagia.

E. This patient has had gastroesophageal reflux disease (GERD) for more than 5 years. Her symptoms are certainly worrisome for cancer. The patient may benefit from a proton pump inhibitor, but evaluation of her dysphagia is most important at this time.

20. | **D.** This patient may have GERD that is manifesting itself as bronchospasm. Specifically, the patient's nighttime symptoms, normal exam, and inability to improve with a metered dose inhaler suggest an extrapulmonary cause for her bronchospasm. GERD may also present with aspiration syndromes, chronic cough, and dental erosions.

A. Long-acting β-agonists are used for treatment in mild-persistent to moderate asthma and may be used in conjunction with inhaled steroids.

B. Inhaled steroids are indicated for patients with mild-persistent to moderate asthma, where symptoms occur more than once a week, but less than once a day.

C. Leukotriene receptor antagonists have been shown to improve baseline function and decreased need for rescue medications in those with moderate asthma.

E. This patient is obviously symptomatic. Additional etiologies for her bronchospasm, such as GERD, should be sought.

21. | **B.** This patient most likely has diverticulitis. Patients with a history of constipation are more likely to have diverticuli that may become inflamed secondary to obstruction of the out-pouching and microperforation leading to local infection. The presentation of diverticulitis includes left lower quadrant pain, fever, nausea, vomiting, and constipation or diarrhea. Plain films should be obtained to rule out free air, ileus, or obstruction. Sigmoidoscopy should not be performed, because this increases risk of perforation. The patient should be placed on antibiotics and IV fluids and made NPO.

A. Inflammatory bowel disease can present with abdominal pain, fever, and stool changes. Often the patient will give you a history of gross blood in the stool and associated weight loss. The onset of inflammatory bowel disease has a bimodal age distribution, with the first peak occurring in the teens and twenties and the second peak occurring around the fifties and sixties.

C. Colon cancer can also present with abdominal pain and change in stool habits. Like inflammatory bowel disease, colon cancer is also associated with weight loss and bloody stool.

D. Diverticulosis is asymptomatic and it describes the herniation of colonic mucosa and submucosa through the colonic wall. A low-fiber diet is thought to contribute to the presence of diverticuli. Diverticulosis can be complicated by bleeding and infection.

E. Appendicitis usually presents with periumbilical pain that then migrates to the right lower quadrant. It is associated with anorexia and usually does not involve pain in the left lower quadrant.

22. | **A.** Diverticulosis and angiodysplasia are the most common causes of lower GI bleeding. The bleeding is thought to occur in the right colon and is secondary to erosion of a diverticular vessel by a fecalith. Patients usually present with sudden onset of cramping with large amounts of hematochezia. Over 90% will stop spontaneously.

B, C, D, E. Hemorrhoids, infectious diarrhea, and inflammatory bowel disease are all causes of lower GI bleeding. Upper GI bleeding accounts for approximately 10% of those episodes initially thought to be considered lower GI bleeds.

23.
> **D.** Infectious esophagitis is the most common cause of odynophagia. *Candida*, cytomegalovirus (CMV), and herpes simplex virus (HSV) are all frequent causes, especially in the immunocompromised patient. Diagnosis is made by biopsy, which shows mucosal inflammation, tissue necrosis, and vascular endothelial involvement. Cytomegalic cells are commonly seen in CMV esophagitis.

A. GERD causes symptoms of heartburn, atypical angina-like pain, and dysphagia. It does not usually cause odynophagia.

B. Achalasia typically presents with a dysphagia for solids *and* liquids. Anatomically, it is secondary to failure of lower esophageal sphincter relaxation. Unlike esophagitis, it does not cause odynophagia. Achalasia can also present with symptoms of GERD.

C. Barrett's esophagus is a precancerous histologic condition in which intestinal columnar epithelium replaces the normal squamous cells in the distal esophagus in response to chronic acid reflux. Barrett's esophagus itself is not symptomatic. Patients will often be symptomatic with heartburn or dysphagia as a result of long-standing GERD.

E. Diffuse esophageal spasm is a motility disorder in which there are simultaneous and repetitive contractions of the esophagus that can present with symptoms of GERD or chest pain. Patients with diffuse esophageal spasm do not normally present with odynophagia, but rather with chest pain that may mimic a myocardial infarction.

24.
> **E.** Eighty percent of gastric carcinomas are attributable to *H. pylori* and seropositivity confers a three- to six-fold risk of gastric cancer. Gastric lymphomas or mucosa-associated lymphoid tissue (MALT) tumors are also thought to be connected to *H. pylori*. Seventy to 80% of gastric lymphomas or MALT tumors will show regression with eradication of *H. pylori*, though it is unknown whether eradication will prevent gastric cancer.

A. Alcohol can promote acid secretion and damage the mucosal barrier, but no evidence suggests that it causes chronic peptic ulcer disease and subsequently gastric adenocarcinoma.

B. NSAID-induced ulcers have no relationship to gastric adenocarcinoma.

C. Tobacco use is most closely associated with lung cancer.

D. Long-standing GERD places a patient at risk for Barrett's esophagus and adenocarcinoma of the esophagus.

25.
> **A.** Gallstones are the most common cause of acute pancreatitis. This patient is also at risk because of her gender, her age, and her obesity. Other causes of pancreatitis include infections (viral and bacterial), hypertriglyceridemia, and hypercalcemia.

B. Alcohol use is the second most common cause of acute pancreatitis and the most common cause of chronic pancreatitis.

C. Trauma can also cause pancreatitis and is seen frequently in children who suffer from blunt abdominal trauma. Pancreatitis after endoscopic retrograde cholangiopancreatography (ERCP) is also a well-known entity. This patient gives no history of trauma.

D. Drugs such as L-asparaginase, Lasix, and didanosine have been known to cause pancreatitis.

E. Tobacco use has no association with pancreatitis.

26.
> **D.** This patient has hemolytic uremic syndrome (HUS), and the likely causative agent is *E. coli* O157:H7. HUS is characterized by a microangiopathic hemolytic anemia, thrombocytopenia, and acute renal failure, and it has a direct correlation to *E. coli* O157:H7. This particular enterohemorrhagic *E. coli* usually causes a bloody diarrhea that may precede the onset of HUS. Renal failure secondary to *E. coli* O157:H7 usually occurs in children aged 5 to 10 years. The organism may be ingested in undercooked beef.

A. *Cryptosporidium* is an intracellular protozoan parasite. Transmission is typically water-borne, but it can also be person to person. It is particularly devastating in the immunocompromised. *Cryptosporidium* is not associated with HUS.

B. *Giardia* is similar to *Cryptosporidium* in that it is a protozoan parasite. Transmission is person-to-person, water-borne, or food-borne. It can present with diarrhea (nonbloody), steatorrhea, malaise, and fatigue, but it is not associated with HUS.

C. Rotavirus is a very common cause of watery, profuse diarrhea in children. It has been associated with intussusception and necrotizing enterocolitis.

E. *Vibrio cholerae* is an enterotoxin-producing, gram-negative bacteria that is water-borne and food-borne. It is very prevalent in Asia and Africa and is known for causing severe dehydration. It is not associated with HUS.

27.
> **B.** In order to meet the Rome Criteria for irritable bowel syndrome, a patient must have abdominal pain that has been present for 12 weeks or more (not necessarily consecutive) in the preceding 12 months. In addition, the pain must have two out of three of the following features: 1) It must be relieved with defecation; 2) Its onset must be associated with a change in the frequency of stooling; 3) Its onset must be associated with a change in appearance (form) of the stool (mucous in the stool is often seen). These symptoms must be in the absence of any structural or metabolic abnormalities which could explain the symptoms, therefore, it is a diagnosis of exclusion.

A. Abdominal pain causing nighttime wakening should be taken more seriously to include problems such as malignancy and vascular disease.

C. Steatorrhea is seen in patients with malabsorption. Causes of malabsorption include pancreatic insufficiency or mucosal abnormalities such as celiac disease.

D. Bloody stool with abdominal pain is a symptom often seen in patients with inflammatory bowel disease, such as Crohn's disease or ulcerative colitis.

E. Weight loss in a patient with abdominal pain and change in stool habits is concerning for malignancy. This patient has had no weight loss and also has no family history of colon cancer.

28. **B.** This man is suffering from acute mesenteric ischemia. The most common cause of acute mesenteric ischemia is arterial embolism. His risk factor is atrial fibrillation that is not appropriately anticoagulated. Presentation is usually acute in nature and the pain is usually out of proportion to the physical exam.

A. Patients with diffuse atherosclerosis will often present with postprandial abdominal pain and early satiety. These changes are more chronic in nature and are sometimes called "intestinal angina."

C. Venous thromboses occur secondary to hypercoagulable states, malignancy, or after trauma or surgery. Patients may present with abdominal pain, and significant bowel edema may be present due to compromised venous drainage. Eventually the arterial circulation may also be compromised, resulting in ischemia. The presentation of mesenteric vein thrombosis is usually not as acute as arterial obstruction from an embolus.

D. Ischemic colitis is secondary to a low-flow state, often a decreased cardiac output. Ischemic colitis can present with abdominal pain, hematochezia, or diarrhea.

E. Small bowel obstruction presents with abdominal pain, nausea, and vomiting. Physical exam is usually significant for abdominal distension and hyperactive bowel sounds, often referred to as "rushing" in nature.

29. **B.** Surgery is the first step in treatment of colon cancer, and it is used not only for excision of the tumor but also for staging when there is not already evidence of metastatic disease on imaging (Dukes class D or stage IV disease). Surgery and pathology can determine the depth of tumor penetration of the mucosa (mucosa and submucosa: Dukes class A; muscularis: Dukes class B1; serosa: Dukes class B2;) and whether there is any lymph node involvement (Dukes class C).

A. Surveillance colonoscopy is not enough, because this patient has pathologic evidence of colon cancer. In a patient with stage I (Dukes class A) colon cancer, or cancer confined to the mucosa, 5-year survival is greater than 90%.

C. Chemotherapy in general is adjunctive therapy and used for palliation. Chemotherapy is given in stage III (Dukes class C) and stage IV (Dukes class D). With chemotherapy and surgery, 5-year survival for stage III is 30% to 60%; for stage IV disease it is less than 5%.

D. Radiation therapy is useful in certain types of rectal cancer but is not indicated in colon cancer.

E. Large-bowel cancers usually spread to the regional lymph nodes or to the liver via the portal circulation first. It rarely spreads to other more distant sites without first being seen in these places, and an MRI of the brain is not indicated at this time for staging because the patient does not have neurologic symptoms and there is no evidence of metastases to the liver or lymph nodes.

30. | **B.** This patient has a first-degree relative with colorectal cancer, so annual fecal occult blood testing is recommended, with sigmoidoscopy every 3 to 5 years or colonoscopy every 10 years, to begin at age 40.

A. There are no recommendations for the general population to begin colonoscopy at age 30.

C. The screening recommendation for the average patient without any risk factors is FOBT annually and sigmoidoscopy every 3 to 5 years or colonoscopy every 10 years, starting at age 50.

D. Patients with a risk of familial adenomatous polyposis should have sigmoidoscopy every 1 to 2 years, starting at age 12.

E. There are no recommendations for FOBT only, without sigmoidoscopy or colonoscopy.

31. | **C.** IVIG has been shown to play a role in treatment of ITP. First-line therapy is high-dose steroids. Over 50% of patients will respond to this treatment with increased platelet counts. Patients who do not respond to high-dose steroids can receive IVIG. Another 60% to 70% of patients respond to this treatment with increased platelet counts. The exact mechanism of IVIG is uncertain, but it appears to inhibit removal of antibody-bound platelets.

A. Peak age of onset for ITP is during childhood between ages 2 and 6; it is usually acute and follows a viral illness. Most children recover spontaneously or require a short course of steroids. Adults with ITP are more likely to experience a chronic and refractory course than children.

B. First-line therapy for ITP is high-dose steroids. Splenectomy is indicated for patients who have been refractory to other treatments and suffer bleeding complications from low platelet counts. All patients should be immunized against *Streptococcus pneumoniae*, *Haemophilus influenzae* type b, and *Neisseria meningitidis* before splenectomy.

D. ITP is caused by IgG and IgM antiplatelet antibodies that attack platelet membrane glycoproteins, leading to platelet destruction.

E. Chronic ITP is defined as persistence of thrombocytopenia for longer than 6 months.

32. **L.** Pyoderma gangrenosum is a skin condition that may be idiopathic or may be associated with systemic disorders such as inflammatory bowel disease (usually ulcerative colitis). It begins as a nodule or hemorrhagic pustule that then breaks down to an ulcer with irregular and raised borders. The ulcer is noninfectious. It is usually treated by treating the underlying disease, but corticosteroids may also be used. The lesion may last months to years.

33. **D.** Acanthosis nigricans is a hyperpigmentation of the skin, occasionally with a velvety appearance. The lesions occur mainly in the axillae, but also other body folds. It is seen in diabetes mellitus and other endocrine disorders; it may also be a paraneoplastic syndrome, primarily associated with adenocarcinoma. The diagnosis is made clinically.

34. **C.** Erythema nodosum is associated with many systemic illnesses, particularly granulomatous diseases. The lesions consist of painful, tender nodules usually on the lower legs but sometimes on the arms. It is frequently seen in sarcoidosis. The diagnosis is clinical and treatment is symptomatic.

35. **G.** Erythema multiforme may be associated with multiple systemic illnesses and may be a reaction to a medication. It is especially common after a herpes simplex viral infection. The lesions consist of target lesions that may be seen on the palms of the hands and soles of the feet. Mucosal involvement may occur. The appearance of the lesions is so characteristic that the diagnosis is usually clinical; the treatment is symptomatic, but corticosteroids may be necessary in severe cases.

36. **A.** Seborrheic dermatitis is a common skin condition characterized by redness of the skin and scaling. The lesions are often greasy. It may involve the scalp and face as well as body folds. The incidence of seborrheic dermatitis is significantly increased in patients with HIV infection. It may be difficult to distinguish from psoriasis. Treatments vary from shampoos containing selenium sulfide to oral ketoconazole. Treatment of the condition when it involves the face can be quite difficult.

37. **H.** Ecthyma gangrenosum results in hemorrhagic bullae that evolve into gangrenous ulcers. It usually occurs in association with *Pseudomonas aeruginosa* bacteremia, primarily in neutropenic or otherwise immunocompromised patients. Diagnosis may be clinical but should be confirmed with biopsy. Treatment is targeted at the underlying bacteremia.

38.   **N.** Erythema migrans is a rash associated with Lyme disease. The lesion is pathognomonic of Lyme disease and consists of a macular, erythematous lesion with central clearing that develops from a macule or papule at the site of the insect bite. The border of the lesion is distinct and red. The lesion may become as large as 15 cm. Most patients have only a solitary lesion, but in a small percentage of patients multiple annular lesions may develop. Treatment targets the underlying Lyme disease.

39.   **M.** Condyloma lata are soft, flat-topped, pale papules and nodules that occur on the genital and perineal skin and are due to secondary syphilis. They are extremely infectious and are similar in appearance to genital warts. Diagnosis is by VDRL, and FTA-ABS may also be positive. Treatment targets the underlying syphilis infection.

40.   **I.** Dermatitis herpetiformis is an intensely pruritic rash that consists of vesicles, papules, and wheals. It usually occurs on the extensor areas of the extremities such as the knees and elbows; it may also occur on the buttocks. It is associated with celiac sprue and/or gluten sensitivity. It may be diagnosed with biopsy. It may be treated with dapsone but is usually completely suppressed by a gluten-free diet.

41.   **K.** Keratoderma blennorrhagicum is a lesion that usually occurs on the feet and consists of papules, vesicles, and pustules. The lesions are usually red to brown and may have a central erosion and become hyperkeratotic. Under the microscope, it looks like psoriasis. The diagnosis of the lesion is mainly clinical. Reactive arthritis and seronegative spondylarthropathy should be ruled out. Treatment is by NSAIDs.

42.   **F.** Porphyria cutanea tarda is associated with hepatitis C, but it may also be idiopathic or secondary to drugs. It consists of vesicles and bullae usually present on the dorsa of the hands. The lesions may occur after minor trauma. Diagnosis is made by biopsy.

B. Cryoglobulins are immunoglobulins and complement that precipitate out of patients' sera and may cause blood vessel damage and inflammation to medium and small vessels. Cryoglobulins are produced in response to infections such as hepatitis C, or they may be a result of hematologic malignancies. They present with palpable purpura of the feet and hands and sometimes ears and tip of the nose.

E. Acute hepatitis B is associated with arthralgia and arthritis due to serum sickness-type immune complex disease. Patients also can have an associated polyarteritis nodosa-type vasculitis.

J. SLE classically presents with a malar rash and photosensitivity as keratinized skin manifestations and as oral aphthous-like ulcers on oral mucous membranes.

43.   **A.** This patient presents with a decline in cognitive function for the past year or so by history of his wife. His past medical history is unremarkable, and he is on no medications, which makes this case relatively simple. He scores an abnormal 24/30 on the screening Mini-Mental State exam, which alerts you to the fact that there is truly a cognitive decline. You need to evaluate for any possible reversible causes of dementia in this patient. The laboratories are normal and, therefore, reassuring in some ways; however, because he has an abnormal "broad-based" gait, you should also be worried about NPH as a diagnosis. This requires a CT scan to evaluate the size of the ventricles in comparison to the cortex. If there is suggestion of NPH, then a removal of a large amount of CSF is done to evaluate for improvement in the balance and cognitive dysfunction. This may help to indicate whether shunting surgery will be beneficial. Our patient had two of the findings in the classic triad for NPH: not every patient will have all three. The triad is: wacky (dementia), wobbly (gait disturbance), and wet (urinary incontinence.)

B. Patients with multi-infarct dementia, also known as vascular dementia, usually have a history of hypertension, hyperlipidemia, and other risk factors for stroke. Often the history will be of sudden, step-like cognitive decline instead of slow, gradual decline that is seen in Alzheimer's and other dementias. Their physical exams usually reveal focal neurologic deficits that are a result of multiple ischemic insults. MRI scan of the brain reveals one or more cerebral infarcts of varying size, or severe diffuse white matter abnormalities. This patient did not present with vascular dementia.

C. Diffuse Lewy-body dementia is now considered the second most common cause of dementia after Alzheimer's disease, accounting for 20% to 25% of dementias. Initial features include impaired attention, concentration, and visuospatial orientation, but often with preserved short-term memory at onset. Patients may have Parkinsonian features of rigidity and cogwheeling and, interestingly, may have sleep disturbances in which they lose the normal REM sleep paralysis and physically act out their dreams while they are asleep.

D. Pick's disease is a type of frontotemporal dementia. The initial most prominent features include personality and behavioral changes with apathy. The Mini-Mental State exam may be normal early in the disease process. CT or MRI of the brain reveals frontal and/or temporal lobe atrophy. Biopsy reveals "Pick bodies," which are cytoplasmic inclusions that stain with silver stain. Clinically, patients may develop hyper-oral behavior, emotional lability, and language disturbance in addition to the dementia.

E. Supranuclear palsy is a degenerative disorder characterized by gliosis, neurofibrillary tangles (different from those in Alzheimer's disease), and neuronal loss in the midbrain, pons, basal ganglia, and cerebellum. Clinically, patients have paresis of voluntary eye movements, specifically downward gaze. Limb rigidity and bradykinesia mimic Parkinson's disease, but there is usually not a tremor. Patients may have frequent falls because of their rigidity and supranuclear ophthalmoplegia. Patients respond poorly to anti-Parkinsonian drugs, and the course is usually progressive, with death occurring within 10 years of diagnosis.

44. **C. Colonoscopy.** Patients who are found to be bacteremic with either *Streptococcus bovis* or *Clostridium septicum* must undergo colonoscopy, because many of them have colon cancer.

A. A transesophageal echocardiogram is more sensitive for detecting infective endocarditis than transthoracic echocardiogram. If the suspicion for infective endocarditis is high and transthoracic echocardiogram is negative, a transesophageal echocardiogram should be performed. However, in this patient, the transthoracic echocardiogram was positive and provided the necessary confirmation of the diagnosis; therefore, transesophageal echocardiogram is not necessary.

B. CT of the abdomen may be helpful in evaluation of the patient's abdominal pain, which may be due to splenic infarction from embolization from his infected heart valve. However, at this time he does not have an acute abdomen and colonoscopy would be more important to rule out cancer.

D. A cardiothoracic surgeon is probably not necessary for this patient at this point. Cardiothoracic surgery evaluation is recommended for patients with infective endocarditis and the following: acute CHF, valve ring abscess, vegetations larger than 1 cm, persistent embolization despite appropriate antibiotic treatment, positive blood cultures despite antibiotic treatment, and first- or second degree heart block.

E. These skin lesions are most likely Janeway lesions in this patient with a high suspicion of infective endocarditis. Therefore, skin biopsy is not necessary. Osler's nodes, also seen in the fingers and toes of patients with infective endocarditis, are nodular and painful, as opposed to Janeway lesions that are macular and painless.

45.

E. 55. This patient has probably had a pulmonary embolism. She is a smoker over the age of 35 and takes oral contraceptives, putting her at risk for venous thromboembolism. The A-a oxygen gradient is the difference between the partial pressure of oxygen in the alveoli and that in the blood. It is often elevated in lung disease that results in ventilation/perfusion mismatch such as pulmonary embolism. The equation for the A-a gradient is as follows:

$$A\text{-}a = pAO_2 - paO_2$$

pAO_2 is the partial pressure of oxygen in the alveoli, and paO_2 is the partial pressure of oxygen in the artery. The value for paO_2 is obtained from the arterial blood gas measurement. The value for pAO_2 is obtained by the following equation:

$$pAO_2 = (FiO_2[\textit{barometric pressure} - \textit{water vapor pressure}]) - (paCO_2/0.8)$$

FiO_2 is the percent of oxygen in inspired air. In the case of room air it is 21% or 0.21. Barometric pressure is 760 mmHg, and water vapor pressure is 47 mmHg at standard conditions. The barometric pressure varies, but for calculations, usually the barometric and water vapor pressures at standard conditions are used. The $paCO_2$ is obtained from the arterial blood gas measurement. The term 0.8 is a respiratory quotient. Under standard conditions, therefore, the equation may be reduced to the following formula.

$$paCO_2 = (0.21)(760 - 47) - (paCO_2/0.8) - paO_2$$
$$= 150 - [paO_2 + (1.25 \times paCO_2)]$$

The normal value for the A-a gradient is 5 to 15 in young patients. The value for the A-a gradient increases with age. This patient's very elevated value of 55 was obtained with the following calculation.

$$paCO_2 = 0.21(760 - 47) - (30/0.8) - 58 = 150 - [58 + (1.25 \times 30)]$$

A,B,C,D. See explanation for E.

46.

E. The patient presented is clinically unstable, as demonstrated by her symptoms (dizziness, shortness of breath) and hypotension. She requires immediate intervention to try to restore her to sinus rhythm. This can be accomplished with medications such as amiodarone, but synchronized cardioversion is faster and the preferred method in an unstable patient requiring immediate intervention.

A, C, D. Whether or not to anticoagulate a patient with atrial fibrillation is an important clinical decision to make. However, this intervention is done to prevent long-term complications of atrial fibrillation, specifically to reduce the incidence of thromboembolic events such as cerebrovascular accidents. It is not the first line of therapy in a patient with unstable atrial fibrillation. Whether to use aspirin or warfarin for long-term prophylaxis depends on various risk factors that must be assessed in each patient, as well on the underlying cause of the atrial fibrillation.

B. Although rate control is the most important initial therapeutic goal in a *stable* patient with atrial fibrillation with rapid ventricular response, the patient described above is *unstable*. Both calcium-channel blockers and β-blockers can be used to suppress AV nodal conduction and subsequently control the rate.

47. **D.** This is a classic presentation of HCM in a young patient. Patients with HCM who are older often present just like patients with valvular aortic stenosis: with angina, syncope (or presyncope) with exertion, or CHF. Fifty percent of patients who present at a younger age have a family history of sudden cardiac death. As the heart rate increases, the filling time of the left ventricle decreases, which decreases the load-dependent cardiac output, resulting in syncope or presyncope.

A. VSDs typically present with dyspnea or are asymptomatic. They rarely present with sudden cardiac death. The murmur associated with VSD is usually holosystolic and located at the left lower sternal border. In addition, although the chest X-ray may be normal, one would expect to see some ventricular enlargement if the VSD were significant enough to cause his symptoms.

B. Pulmonary embolus may present as sudden cardiac death, but not usually in healthy, younger patients (unless there is an underlying hypercoagulable state present). In addition, a pulmonary embolus does not produce the murmur noted on his exam. There are a variety of chest X-ray findings that can be seen with a pulmonary embolus, one of which is a normal chest X-ray.

C. Tension pneumothorax is certainly a consideration for sudden collapse in a tall, thin, otherwise healthy patient. However, his chest X-ray would have revealed evidence of this, and it did not.

E. An aortic dissection is uncommon in healthy young people. Also, the murmur heard on his exam was not consistent with an aortic aneurysm. Again, one would expect to see changes on his chest X-ray such as widening of the mediastinum, which was not noted.

48. **B.** This case illustrates classic findings of coarctation of the aorta. Patients who have coarctation often present with progressive symptoms of fatigue and dyspnea. Although the diagnosis is usually made in childhood, it is occasionally not made until early adulthood. Due to the location of the narrowing, or coarctation, in the descending aorta, the arteries supplying the upper extremities and chest experience a high back pressure, whereas the arterial supply to the lower extremities remains relatively normal or diminished. This explains the typical finding of isolated upper extremity hypertension and often diminished pulses in the lower extremities. The elevated blood pressure within the intercostal arteries account for the rib notching seen on chest X-ray.

A. ASDs often result in a left-to-right shunt, which lead to increased pressures within the right side of the heart. This ultimately leads to right ventricular enlargement that can sometimes be seen on chest X-ray in addition to "shunt vascularity." The ECG finding with ASD is usually right-axis deviation with or without right-bundle branch block, not usually LVH. In addition, the ASD does not usually result in hypertension.

C. AS occurs proximal to the arteries supplying the upper extremities and chest, and subsequently does not result in upper extremity hypertension and rib notching on chest X-ray. Although the murmur of AS is often midsystolic, it is usually best heard at the right upper sternal border with radiation into the carotid arteries, not the back.

D. PDA produces a continuous murmur that is heard throughout systole and diastole. In addition, PDA does not cause rib notching and hypertension. Calcification of the ductus arteriosus is the classic finding of PDA on chest X-ray.

E. HCM involves the intraventricular septum and does not cause isolated upper extremity hypertension. Although it can cause LVH, it does not account for the rib notching seen on chest X-ray.

49.

> **A.** The murmur of HCM is the result of turbulent flow through the narrowing of the left ventricular outflow tract. This narrowing is caused by hypertrophy of the intraventricular septum and the anterior motion of the mitral valve leaflets that occur during systole. As blood flow through this area decreases, the intraventricular septum is allowed to move closer to the mitral leaflets, making the outlet narrower. This in turn makes the murmur louder. Conversely, as flow across this narrowing increases, the septum is pushed further away from the mitral leaflets resulting in a wider outlet, decreased turbulence and a softer murmur. The Valsalva maneuver increases intrathoracic pressure and subsequently decreases venous return to the heart. As a result, there is less blood to fill the ventricle, allowing the obstruction to worsen and the murmur to become louder.

B. AS results in a valve that has a relatively fixed obstruction. The Valsalva maneuver decreases venous return to the heart. Subsequently, as blood flow across this tight, stenotic valve decreases, so does the amount of turbulence; the murmur of AS thus becomes softer.

C. The murmur of AI is the result of retrograde blood flow across the aortic valve that occurs during diastole. Because the Valsalva increases intrathoracic pressure and decreases venous return to the heart, it causes less blood to flow back across the aortic valve into the heart, making the murmur softer.

D. The relationship between blood flow and turbulence across a stenotic mitral valve is similar to that of AS. As flow across the valve decreases, so does the murmur. Therefore, the murmur of mitral stenosis is made softer with the Valsalva maneuver.

E. Again, the relationship between the murmur and the flow across a stenotic tricuspid valve is no different than that outlined for the stenotic aortic or mitral valves. Therefore, by decreasing venous return to the heart and ultimately decreasing flow across the valve, the Valsalva maneuver makes the murmur of tricuspid stenosis softer.

50. | **C.** The above markers are released from the myocyte during injury or death, which is often the result of an acute myocardial infarction. The rates at which they rise, peak, and return to normal are all different. Myoglobin is the first to become elevated at 1 to 4 hours and the first to peak at 6 to 7 hours. Myoglobin's peak is followed, in order, by CPK-MB, troponin-I, and LDH. The order in which they return to baseline differs, however. Myoglobin is the first to return to baseline, followed by CPK-MB, and then LDH. Troponin-I remains elevated for up to 10 to 12 days after an acute myocardial infarction.

A, B, D, E. See explanation for C.

Questions

> **The next two questions (items 51 and 52) correspond to the following vignette.**

An otherwise healthy 31-year-old woman presents with complaints of new-onset substernal chest pain. She states the pain is persistent, worse with inspiration, and improved by leaning forward. She states she has had subjective fevers for the past 2 days. On exam, she has normal vital signs and is afebrile. She appears uncomfortable, but is in no acute distress. Her lungs are clear to auscultation and you think you hear a faint friction rub. Chest X-ray is normal. You obtain the following ECG (Figure 51).

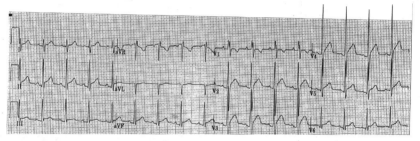

Figure 51 • Image courtesy of Dr. Brenda Shinar, Banner Good Samaritan Medical Center, Phoenix, Arizona

51. What is the diagnosis?

    A. Pulmonary embolus
    B. Acute myocardial infarction
    C. Pericarditis
    D. Tension pneumothorax
    E. Cardiac tamponade

52. What is the initial treatment of choice for this patient?

    A. Anticoagulation with IV heparin
    B. Treatment with β-blockers
    C. Initiation of anti-inflammatory medication
    D. Thoracostomy with placement of chest tube
    E. Pericardiocentesis with placement of pericardial window

End of set

> **The response options for items 53 through 58 are the same. You will be required to select one answer for each item in the set.**

    A. Aortic stenosis (AS)
    B. Aortic regurgitation
    C. Mitral stenosis
    D. Mitral regurgitation
    E. Tricuspid stenosis
    F. Tricuspid regurgitation
    G. Patent ductus arteriosus (PDA)
    H. Coarctation of the aorta

For each description, select the appropriate murmur.

53. Diastolic rumbling murmur with opening snap heard best in the area of the apex.

54. High-pitched, decrescendo mid- to holodiastolic murmur heard at the third and fourth intercostal space at the left sternal border.

55. Diastolic murmur heard best at the left lower sternal border.

56. Diamond-shaped systolic ejection murmur heard at the right upper sternal border.

57. Pansystolic decrescendo murmur heard best at the apex with radiation into the axilla.

58. Systolic murmur heard best at the left lower sternal border that increases with inspiration.

End of set

> **The next two questions (items 59 and 60) correspond to the following vignette.**

A 70-year-old man with long-standing hypertension presents to the ED with complaints of acute onset of substernal chest pain. He describes the pain as "tearing" in nature with radiation into his back. On exam, his blood pressure is 172/102 with a pulse of 118. He appears uncomfortable and diaphoretic. His cardiac exam reveals tachycardia with a normal S_1 and S_2. There are no murmurs noted. You suspect an aortic dissection.

59. Which of the following would be the test of choice to confirm your diagnosis?

    A. ECG
    B. Chest X-ray
    C. Transesophageal echocardiogram (TEE)
    D. Transthoracic echocardiogram (TTE)
    E. CT scan of the chest

60. The above test confirms the presence of a 7-cm ascending thoracic aortic dissection. Your first step in the initial therapeutic management of this patient is to:

    A. Transfuse platelets and fresh-frozen plasma.
    B. Treat with IV β-blockers and nitroprusside
    C. Obtain a cardiothoracic surgery consult
    D. Observe the patient and perform serial echocardiograms
    E. Treat with oral angiotensin-converting enzyme (ACE) inhibitors

End of set

---

61. You have just started your hematology-oncology rotation and you are seeing a patient in the clinic for follow-up of breast cancer treatment. She is frightened about her diagnosis and asks you questions regarding mortality from breast cancer and other kinds of cancers. You counsel her that which of the following cancers is responsible for the most cancer-related deaths in women in the United States per year?

    A. Colorectal cancer
    B. Lung cancer
    C. Breast cancer
    D. Leukemia
    E. Ovarian cancer

The next two questions (items 62 and 63) correspond to the following vignette.

A 25-year-old Hispanic woman presents to your office after finding a lump in her left breast. She found the lump when taking a shower 3 months ago and has not noticed any change in the size or consistency of the lump with her menstrual cycles. She has no significant medical history and takes no medications. She began menses at age 10 and gave birth to a son at age 21. Family history is significant for a paternal aunt with breast cancer. On physical exam there is a palpable mass in the left upper outer quadrant of the left breast. It is approximately 3 cm in diameter, smooth, and well circumscribed. No axillary nodes are palpable.

62. The next step in evaluating this patient should be:

    A. Excisional biopsy
    B. Mammogram
    C. Ultrasound
    D. Mastectomy
    E. Reassurance and follow-up in 6 months

63. Which of the following is a risk factor for breast cancer in this patient?

    A. Personal history of breast cancer
    B. First-degree relative with breast cancer
    C. Race
    D. Age at menarche
    E. Age at first live birth

End of set

The next two questions (items 64 and 65) correspond to the following vignette.

A 34-year-old white man presents with a complaint of blood in his bowel movements for the last 2 weeks. He also has noted some symptoms of constipation and change in stool caliber. He does not report any weight loss, fatigue, or emesis. He has noted a mild decrease in appetite. His family history is positive for a father with colon cancer diagnosed at age 50, a female sibling with colon cancer diagnosed at age 45, and an aunt with colon cancer diagnosed at age 54. A colonoscopy is performed with biopsy of a single ulcerative mass in the descending colon. The pathology shows adenocarcinoma.

64. Which genetic condition do you suspect in this patient?

    A. Familial adenomatous polyposis (FAP)

    B. BRCA-1 mutation

    C. Gardner's syndrome

    D. Hereditary nonpolyposis colorectal cancer (HNPCC)

    E. Peutz-Jeghers syndrome

65. What recommendations do you have for screening this patient's other family members?

    A. One stool guaiac card per day for three consecutive days done annually starting at age 15 for all family members

    B. Colonoscopy for all family members starting at age 20 or 10 years younger than the age at which the youngest family member was diagnosed with colon cancer, whichever comes first

    C. Female family members should abide by the usual screening rules for gynecologic cancers

    D. Colonoscopy for all family members at age 30, and if it is normal, repeat every 10 years

    E. Flexible sigmoidoscopy for all family members when they are 10 years younger than the age at which the youngest family member was diagnosed with colon cancer

End of set

---

66. A 76-year-old man presents to your office with a complaint of hemoptysis for 1 week. He states that he coughs up about a teaspoon of blood a couple of times a day. He denies fever or purulent sputum. He also reports a weight loss of 10 pounds over the last month and increasing dyspnea. He has a cigarette smoking history of 60 pack/years. Physical exam does not reveal any abnormalities on cardiovascular or pulmonary examination. Chest X-ray shows mediastinal enlargement, and CT shows a perihilar mass and significant lymphadenopathy. Bronchoscopy is performed, and biopsies of the mass are taken. The pathology reveals islands of small, round, deeply basophilic-staining epithelial cells that look like lymphocytes, but are about twice the size of normal lymphocytes. Which of the following statements is true regarding his disease?

    A. Untreated patients with his disease have median survival rates of 12 to 14 months

    B. Surgery is a mainstay of treatment

    C. Subacute cortical cerebellar degeneration is a paraneoplastic syndrome associated with his disease

    D. His disease is not associated with his tobacco use

    E. The tumor arises from type II pneumocytes in the alveolar wall

---

The response options for items 67 through 69 are the same. You will be required to select one answer for each item in the set.

    A. Human T-cell lymphotrophic virus-1 (HTLV-1)
    B. Epstein-Barr virus (EBV)
    C. *Helicobacter pylori*
    D. Cytomegalovirus (CMV)
    E. Human herpesvirus 8 (HHV-8)

For each lymphoma, select the associated infection.

67. Burkitt's lymphoma

68. Mucosa-associated lymphoid tissue (MALT) lymphoma

69. Adult T-cell lymphoma

End of set

---

70. A 60-year-old man with an 80 pack-year history of smoking presents with a complaint of "turning yellow" over the last 2 weeks. He reports nausea, but no vomiting or abdominal pain. He has no other significant medical history and no history of alcohol abuse. He notes a decrease in his appetite over the last month, a 5-pound weight loss, and a slight increase in abdominal girth. On physical exam, the vitals signs are within normal limits. His skin is visibly jaundiced, and his sclerae are icteric. The exam otherwise reveals a minimally distended, nontender abdomen. Labs reveal the following: WBC 6000/μL with normal differential; hemoglobin 11.8 g/dL; blood smear normal; total bilirubin 13.0 mg/dL; direct bilirubin 11.5 mg/dL; indirect bilirubin 1.5 mg/dL; AST 45 U/L; ALT 55 U/L; alkaline phosphatase 200 U/L. What is the most likely diagnosis?

    A. Cholecystitis
    B. Pancreatic cancer
    C. Ascending cholangitis
    D. Gilbert's syndrome
    E. Autoimmune hemolytic anemia

71. A 70-year-old man presents with bone pain in his lower back and pelvis bilaterally for the past 2 weeks. He has been increasingly fatigued over the last 2 months. He denies weight loss, night sweats, easy bruising, or bleeding. He has been to an urgent care for upper respiratory infections twice in the last 3 months. On physical examination you note spinous process tenderness to palpation over the lumbar vertebrae and tenderness of the pelvis and long bones of the thighs. Otherwise examination is unremarkable. Labs are as follows: Hemoglobin 8.9 g/dL; WBCs 5000/μL; platelets 300,000/μL; creatinine 1.9 mg/dL; calcium 11.2 mg/dL; total protein 9.1 g/dL. The remainder of electrolytes and liver function tests are normal. What is the most likely diagnosis?

    A. Acute lymphocytic leukemia
    B. Monoclonal gammopathy of unknown significance (MGUS)
    C. Waldenström's macroglobulinemia
    D. Chronic myelogenous leukemia
    E. Multiple myeloma

72. A 20-year-old man presents with shortness of breath for the last 6 weeks. He complains of dyspnea on exertion, palpitations, weight loss of 15 pounds, fever, and night sweats. On examination his pulse is 120, respiratory rate 18, and oxygen saturations are 98% on room air. A fixed, firm, 3-cm left anterior cervical lymph node is palpable. Lungs are clear to auscultation bilaterally, and the patient has no enlargement of the liver or spleen. The remainder of the exam is normal. A chest X-ray shows mediastinal lymphadenopathy. Excisional biopsy of the cervical lymph node reveals cells seen in Figure 72. What is his most likely diagnosis?

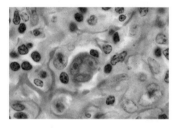

Figure 72 • Image courtesy of Dr. Brenda Shinar, Banner Good Samaritan Medical Center, Phoenix, Arizona

A. CMV
B. Hodgkin's lymphoma
C. Non-Hodgkin's lymphoma
D. Scrofula
E. Sarcoidosis

73. A 75-year-old man with small cell carcinoma presents with shortness of breath, facial swelling, and headache. On physical exam respiratory rate is 18, his oxygen saturation is 94% on room air and he is not in any acute distress. There is cervical venous distension, plethora of the face, and facial edema. You suspect superior vena cava (SVC) syndrome. Which of the following statements is true regarding this diagnosis?

A. Lymphoma is the most common cause of SVC syndrome
B. Stridor due to tracheal obstruction is a medical emergency and should be treated immediately with radiation
C. The most common physical finding is facial edema
D. Symptoms can be decreased by elevating the head of the bed, providing oxygen, and gentle diuresis
E. Radiation therapy has no effect on prognosis

74. You are asked to design a screening test for disease "X." Knowing that approximately 20% of the general population has disease "X," you develop a screening test, which you use on 1000 randomly selected patients. The following numbers are obtained: People *with* disease and a positive screening test, 180; people *without* disease and *with* a positive screening test, 160; people *with* disease and a negative screening test, 20; people *without* disease and *with* a negative screening test, 640. Which of the following statements regarding the screening test is true?

A. The specificity is 90%
B. The specificity is 60%
C. The sensitivity is 40%
D. The sensitivity is 66%
E. The sensitivity is 90%

The next two questions (items 75 and 76) correspond to the following vignette.

A 28-year-old man presents to the ED with complaints of abdominal pain, nausea, and vomiting. He has had three episodes of emesis over the past 24 hours. His abdominal pain is localized to the epigastric and right upper quadrant areas. He has had no diarrhea. He reports increasing jaundice, but denies dark urine or light-colored stools. He has had no recent travel. On examination, he is afebrile and has normal vital signs. He is in no acute distress, but obviously does not feel well. He has mild scleral and mucosal icterus, but the remainder of his head and neck exam is unremarkable. His lungs are clear, and his heart examination is normal. He has diffuse abdominal tenderness that is worse in the right upper quadrant area. His abdomen is not distended. He has no rebound, guarding, or rigidity. His genitourinary (GU) examination is normal and stool is negative for occult blood. You obtain the following laboratory results: AST 4800 U/L; ALT 3900 U/L; total bilirubin 2.1 mg/dL; alkaline phosphatase 152 U/L; PT 12.6 seconds.

75. What is the most likely cause of this patient's clinical presentation?

   A. Viral hepatitis
   B. Cholelithiasis
   C. Alcoholic hepatitis
   D. Hemochromatosis
   E. Hepatocellular carcinoma

76. What is the next appropriate test to obtain on this patient?

   A. Abdominal ultrasound
   B. Ethanol level
   C. Percutaneous liver biopsy
   D. Percentage of transferrin saturated with iron (also known as % sat)
   E. Acute hepatitis panel

End of set

---

77. A 54-year-old man presents to your office for a pre-employment physical. He is currently treated for allergic rhinitis with a steroid preparation nasal spray, but is otherwise healthy and takes no other medications. He offers no specific complaints during his visit. He drinks infrequently and smokes approximately two packs of cigarettes per day for the past 10 years. His physical examination is normal, including his vital signs. He gives you some papers from his employer to complete regarding his physical exam and health status. The forms include a request for an ECG, a chest X-ray, and some routine labs. You order these as requested. His ECG is normal as are his routine labs. You receive a report that his chest X-ray reveals a single, round lesion near the periphery of his right upper lobe. It is approximately 2 cm in diameter and is surrounded by normal lung parenchyma. There is no evidence of lymphadenopathy on the chest X-ray. There are no old chest X-rays available for comparison. You obtain a CT scan of his chest, which confirms the presence of an eccentric 2-cm lesion in the right upper lobe near the chest wall. Which of the following is the most appropriate next step in the management of this patient?

A. Have him follow up in 3 months for a repeat chest X-ray
B. Have him follow up in 6 months for a repeat chest X-ray
C. Make arrangements for him to have a CT-guided needle biopsy of the lesion
D. Make arrangements for him to have a bronchoscopy with transbronchial biopsies of the lesion
E. Apply a PPD and start empiric therapy for tuberculosis

78. A 72-year-old woman presents to the ED with a severe exacerbation of her chronic obstructive pulmonary disease (COPD). She is in respiratory distress and requires immediate intubation and placement on a mechanical ventilator. Once she is stabilized, she is admitted to the intensive care unit where you are working. A nurse asks you about the possibility of her developing a deep venous thrombosis (DVT) and possible pulmonary embolism (PE). Which of the following statements is correct regarding the prevention of venous thromboembolism (VTE) in this patient?

A. She is at low risk for VTE and does not need prophylaxis
B. 5000 U of subcutaneous heparin should be given every 8 to 12 hours
C. Sequential compression devices (SCDs) should be applied to her lower extremities
D. Full dose IV heparin should be initiated
E. She should be evaluated for a hypercoagulable state before beginning DVT prophylaxis

79. You are rotating in the intensive care unit and taking care of several patients. On rounds, your attending asks you to choose which one out of five of your patients is at the highest risk for the development of a stress ulcer complication. Your choice is:

A. A 62-year-old woman on a mechanical ventilator because of severe COPD exacerbation
B. A 58-year-old man who is on IV heparin therapy for an acute myocardial infarction
C. A 60-year-old woman with acute pancreatitis with a prior history of upper GI bleed
D. A 55-year-old man with COPD and a large pulmonary embolus who developed respiratory failure requiring ventilation and is on IV heparin therapy
E. A woman with rheumatoid arthritis with a septic knee and hypotension

80. A 62-year-old woman presents to your office complaining of a cough that has been present for the past 8 weeks. She says the cough is nonproductive and is not associated with fevers or shortness of breath. There is no history of tobacco use. She has not noticed the cough being worse at night, but does report it seems worse when she lies flat. She has hypertension that is well controlled with a β-blocker, but has been healthy otherwise. She has no history of asthma and denies wheezing with this cough or any recent respiratory tract infections. There is no history of seasonal allergy symptoms. There are no identifiable risk factors for tuberculosis. She states that she has fairly frequent heartburn but denies weight loss or dysphagia. Her vital signs are normal and she is afebrile. Her physical examination is completely normal. What is the most likely cause of her chronic cough?

A. Seasonal allergies
B. Postnasal drip
C. Gastroesophageal reflux
D. Asthma variant
E. Bronchogenic carcinoma

81. A 58-year-old man, accompanied by his wife, presents to your office with complaints of progressive difficulty swallowing. He has a sensation of the food getting "stuck" in his chest. He says that the difficulty swallowing first started with breads and meats a few months ago and now occurs with most foods. He has no trouble swallowing liquids. He denies any nausea or vomiting. He does not choke on his food or have any difficulty chewing or initiating a swallow. His wife confirms this and states she believes he has lost approximately 15 pounds over the past 4 months. His past medical history is significant only for hypertension, which is well controlled. He reports chronic reflux-type symptoms that he treats with over-the-counter antacids. He is not a smoker. His vital signs are normal, and his physical examination is unremarkable. An ECG and chest X-ray are obtained, both of which are normal. What is the most likely diagnosis and the best test to evaluate for it?

    A. Achalasia; upper GI barium study
    B. Diverticulum; CT scan
    C. Adenocarcinoma: esophagogastroduodenoscopy (EGD)
    D. Squamous cell carcinoma: EGD
    E. Candidiasis; candida skin testing

The next two questions (items 82 and 83) correspond to the following vignette.

A 26-year-old white woman comes to your office after noticing a lump in her breast approximately 1 week ago. She states that she had never noticed it before. She is fearful because her grandmother had breast cancer diagnosed at age 75. She notes that the lump is tender and moveable. She does not recall any trauma to the area. She is due for her period in 2 weeks. On exam you note a smooth, round, 1.5-cm mass that is fluctuant and minimally tender.

82. What is the most likely diagnosis?

    A. Breast adenocarcinoma
    B. Fibrous adenoma
    C. Breast abscess
    D. Fat necrosis
    E. Breast cyst

83. You have advised her to observe the mass throughout her menses and return if it does not go away. She returns 2 weeks later and is concerned that the mass is still present and is, in fact, larger. On exam it has grown to 2 cm in size but still remains smooth, round and fluctuant. The next diagnostic step is:

    A. BRCA-1 and BRCA-2 gene testing
    B. Ultrasound
    C. Mammogram
    D. Surgical referral for excision
    E. Wait and reexamine in 3 months

End of set

84. A 19-year-old white woman presents to your office with complaints of irregular periods. She states she has had irregular periods since menarche at age 14. Her periods occur every 28 to 40 days and last 4 to 5 days. It has been approximately 60 days since her last period. She is very athletic and plays basketball on her college team. Her weight has been stable without any recent extreme losses or gains. She states she is currently sexually active but states she and her boyfriend always use condoms. Her BMI is 25, and her physical exam, including pelvic exam, is within normal limits. What should you do next to evaluate the cause of her irregular periods?

    A. Start a low estrogen/progestin oral contraceptive pill to regulate her cycle
    B. Get a urine β-HCG to rule out pregnancy
    C. Recommend that she check daily basal body temperatures to evaluate for ovulation
    D. Order a TSH
    E. Refer for an endometrial biopsy

85. A 55-year-old white woman with a history of hypertension presents to your office with complaints of a red right eye. She states that she noticed it approximately 2 days ago. She denies any recent viral illness or eye discharge. She is very uncomfortable with a deep, severe aching pain behind her right eye that she has never felt before. She had associated nausea and vomiting today secondary to the severe pain. On physical exam, the eye is diffusely erythematous without discharge. The cornea appears cloudy. The pupil is moderately dilated and fixed, without a response to light. The vision in the affected eye is markedly blurred. What is the most likely diagnosis?

    A. Viral conjunctivitis
    B. Herpes simplex keratitis
    C. Corneal abrasion
    D. Acute angle-closure glaucoma
    E. Allergic conjunctivitis

86. A 28-year-old Hispanic woman comes to your office for a routine health exam. She states she has not had a Pap and pelvic exam in 6 years. She is currently sexually active, and has been in a monogamous relationship for 4 years. She has had a total of two sexual partners starting at age 20. She denies alcohol, tobacco, or IV drug abuse (IVDA). Her exam, including pelvic, is within normal limits. You obtain her Pap results and it reveals atypical squamous cells of unknown significance (ASCUS). What do you do next in the management of this patient?

    A. Repeat Pap and pelvic in 1 year and repeat yearly until three are consecutively negative
    B. Refer for colposcopy with biopsy
    C. Human papilloma virus (HPV) gene typing
    D. Refer for colposcopy with cryotherapy
    E. Repeat Pap and pelvic every 4 to 6 months until three are consecutively negative

87. A 60-year-old white man presents to your office for a new patient visit. He states that in general he is fairly healthy with the exception of hypertension for which he is taking hydrochlorothiazide. On review of systems, his only concern is that his last doctor told him that he had blood in his stool when checked in the office and that he would need follow-up. He was unable to do this at that time because he lost his insurance. He denies any weight loss or change in appetite. He also denies any change in stools. He denies any family history of colorectal cancer. Exam reveals internal hemorrhoids. Repeat fecal occult blood test is positive. The next step in his evaluation is:

A. Single contrast barium enema
B. Anoscopy, to evaluate the hemorrhoids for bleeding
C. Flexible sigmoidoscopy
D. Colonoscopy
E. CT scan of abdomen and pelvis

The response options for items 88 through 91 are the same. You will be required to select one answer for each item in the set.

A. Intrauterine device (IUD)
B. Progestin only, injection form
C. Combination oral contraceptive pill (OCP) (estrogen/progesterone)
D. Condom

For each description, select the appropriate form of contraceptive.

88. Inhibits ovulation by suppressing follicle-stimulating hormone (FSH) and luteinizing hormone (LH). Success is determined by taking this medication consistently.

89. Long-term suppression of ovulation, often used in adolescents. Side effects include irregular uterine bleeding, headache, breast tenderness, weight gain, and acne.

90. Progesterone-containing device associated with an increased risk of pelvic inflammatory disease (PID) in high-risk patients, such as those with multiple sex partners or with a history of sexually transmitted diseases (STDs). Side effects include increased uterine cramping and bleeding.

91. When used with spermicide it is associated with increased effectiveness. Is also associated with a decreased transmission of STDs.

End of set

The next two questions (items 92 and 93) correspond to the following vignette.

A 20-year-old white woman presents to your office with a 3- to 4-day history of dysuria and increased frequency of urination. She denies fever, chills, or flank pain. She is currently sexually active with her boyfriend. She states they use condoms all of the time. She has recently noted a vaginal discharge that has an unusual odor. Urine dip in the office is negative. On pelvic exam you note a thin, white vaginal discharge adhering to the vaginal wall. The cervix is otherwise within normal limits. There is no cervical motion tenderness. The pH of the vaginal discharge is 6. A wet mount preparation reveals epithelial cells that are covered with coccobacillary bacteria, which makes the cells appear stippled.

92. What is the most likely diagnosis?

- **A.** Urinary tract infection with *E. coli*
- **B.** Bacterial vaginosis
- **C.** *Trichomonas* infection
- **D.** *Chlamydia trachomatis* infection
- **E.** Vulvovaginal candidiasis

93. The most appropriate therapy for bacterial vaginosis is:

- **A.** Trimethoprim-sulfamethoxazole
- **B.** Ciprofloxacin
- **C.** Metronidazole
- **D.** Diflucan
- **E.** Ceftriaxone

End of set

---

94. A 55-year-old obese man comes to your office with concerns regarding diabetes. His mother and father both suffer from diabetes type II, diagnosed in their adult years. He denies any history of polyuria or polydipsia. His past medical history is significant only for hypertension, for which he is trying diet and exercise with little success. His body mass index (BMI) is 40, heart rate 90, respiratory rate 18, and blood pressure 149/79. Exam is significant for an obese man with noted acanthosis nigricans. You suspect he has type II diabetes mellitus and you order laboratories. Which of the following would be consistent with a diagnosis of diabetes?

- **A.** Random glucose >180
- **B.** Postprandial 2-hour plasma glucose >120
- **C.** HgbA1C of 7.0
- **D.** Fasting glucose >126
- **E.** + glucose on urine dipstick

95. A 56-year-old white woman presents to you with complaints of urinary incontinence. She notes that she senses an intense need to use the bathroom but often does not make it to the bathroom on time. She is not incontinent with coughing or sneezing. She denies any dysuria, fevers, or abdominal pain. She is not currently taking any medications. She is incontinent two or three times per week. Physical exam is essentially within normal limits. Urinalysis is within normal limits and postvoid residual is <40 mL. This patient's symptoms best fit which category of incontinence?

    A. Overflow and urge incontinence
    B. Overflow and stress incontinence
    C. Urge incontinence
    D. Stress incontinence
    E. Overflow incontinence

The next three questions (items 96 through 98) correspond to the following vignette.

A 41-year-old man with diabetes mellitus presents with a cough associated with pleuritic chest pain, which began yesterday. His cough is productive of thick, rust-colored sputum. He has been having fevers up to 103.0°F (39.4°C) and shaking chills. On examination, you find a well-developed man with temperature 102.6°F (39.2°C), blood pressure 118/68, heart rate 98, and respiratory rate 24. Room air pulse-oximetry reveals an oxygen saturation of 86% that increases to 94% on 2 L/min nasal cannula. His lung exam reveals bronchial breath sounds in his right lower lung base with egophony. His heart rate is mildly tachycardic without murmur or ectopy noted. Abdominal and GU exam is normal. A CBC reveals a WBC count of 18,400 with a left shift. His chest X-ray demonstrates a focal, consolidative infiltrate in the right lower lobe area with an associated pleural effusion.

96. Which of the following organisms has most likely caused his presentation?

    A. *Mycoplasma pneumoniae*
    B. *Pneumocystis carinii*
    C. *Bacteroides fragilis*
    D. *Streptococcus pneumoniae*
    E. *Bacillus anthracis*

97. Which of the following antibiotics would be the best choice for initial therapy of his infection?

    A. Clindamycin
    B. Ceftriaxone
    C. Sulfamethoxazole-trimethoprim
    D. Ampicillin
    E. Amantadine

98. You perform a thoracentesis to obtain fluid to evaluate this patient's new pleural effusion. A simultaneous serum sample is drawn and shows a total protein (TP) level of 6.5 and an LDH level of 220. Which of the following are you most likely to find on his pleural fluid analysis (Table 98)?

Answer	Effusion Total Protein (TP)	Effusion LDH
■ TABLE 98		
A.	4.0	180
B.	3.0	60
C.	2.5	80
D.	2.0	100
E.	1.0	120

End of set

The next two questions (items 99 and 100) correspond to the following vignette.

A 31-year-old man presents to the ED with complaints of a painful, swollen right index finger. He states that the onset of swelling and pain started the day before. Other than a subjective fever and malaise, he has no other complaints. On review of systems, he reports some mild dysuria which began approximately 2 weeks ago. He denies penile discharge. He has had several female sexual partners over the past few months. He denies any GI complaints or skin rashes. On examination, he is afebrile and his vital signs are normal. He has mild erythema of the conjunctiva of the right eye without photophobia. The remainder of his examination is unremarkable with the exception of his right index finger (Figure 99).

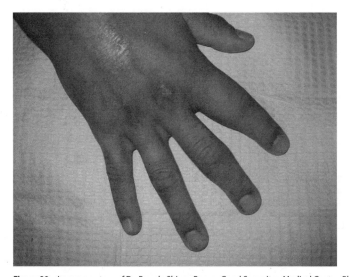

Figure 99 • Image courtesy of Dr. Brenda Shinar, Banner Good Samaritan Medical Center, Phoenix, Arizona

99. What is the most likely cause of this patient's symptoms?

    A. Psoriatic arthritis
    B. Rheumatoid arthritis
    C. Reiter's syndrome
    D. Gonococcal arthritis
    E. Osteoarthritis

100. Which of the following is most likely to be positive in this patient?

    A. Culture of joint aspirate
    B. Rheumatoid factor
    C. Urethral DNA probe for gonorrhea
    D. HLA-B27
    E. Plain film periosteal elevation and thickening

End of set

51.	C	68.	C	85.	D
52.	C	69.	A	86.	C
53.	C	70.	B	87.	D
54.	B	71.	E	88.	C
55.	E	72.	B	89.	B
56.	A	73.	D	90.	A
57.	D	74.	E	91.	D
58.	F	75.	A	92.	B
59.	E	76.	E	93.	C
60.	B	77.	C	94.	D
61.	B	78.	B	95.	C
62.	C	79.	D	96.	D
63.	D	80.	C	97.	B
64.	D	81.	C	98.	A
65.	B	82.	E	99.	C
66.	C	83.	B	100.	D
67.	B	84.	B		

51. C. This patient has classic findings of pericarditis. These include pleuritic chest pain that is affected by positioning, fevers, and a friction rub. The ECG shows diffuse ST segment elevation that is suggestive of a global process, and PR depression.

A. Although a pulmonary embolus can cause substernal chest pain and fever in a young woman, the pain is usually not affected by positioning. In addition, the ECG findings most often show sinus tachycardia with or without evidence of right-sided heart strain.

B. Acute myocardial infarction would be an unusual cause of chest pain in a young patient. Pain resulting from myocardial ischemia does not usually have a pleuritic component to it. In addition, one would not expect to see diffuse ST segment changes on the ECG, but rather a specific pattern of injury (for example, leads II, III, and AVF would be affected in an inferior wall myocardial infarction).

D. Tension pneumothorax could also cause pleuritic chest pain in a young patient, but it is not usually affected by positioning. Additionally, it would not account for the ECG changes shown, and one would not expect to see a normal chest X-ray.

E. Cardiac tamponade does not usually present with chest pain, but rather with dyspnea and symptoms similar to those of congestive heart failure, such as orthopnea and lower extremity edema. However, patients in tamponade should have clear lung fields on auscultation, which distinguishes them from patients in left heart failure. In addition, tamponade does not usually cause diffuse ST-segment elevation on ECG, but rather low voltage throughout all the leads. This is due to the dampening of the electrical impulse as it traverses the fluid surrounding the heart.

52. C. The patient with pericarditis should be started initially on anti-inflammatory medications such as aspirin or NSAIDs. For refractory cases of pericarditis, other medications such as colchicine or steroids may be indicated.

A. The treatment of choice for a pulmonary embolus would be to initiate anticoagulation with IV heparin. However, this is contraindicated in a patient with pericarditis because of the increased risk of bleeding from the inflamed pericardium, which could lead to a hemorrhagic effusion and tamponade.

B. Although β-blockers would be indicated if she were having an acute myocardial infarction, they are of no benefit in the treatment of pericarditis.

D. Thoracostomy with placement of chest tube would be helpful in a patient with a pneumothorax. However, it will be of no benefit to our patient.

E. Pericardiocentesis with placement of pericardial window may be indicated in some cases of cardiac tamponade; however, it is of no benefit in the treatment of pericarditis without pericardial effusion. An echocardiogram will help you determine whether or not a pericardial effusion is present.

53. C. The murmur of mitral stenosis is best heard in the area of the mitral valve (the apex) and occurs during diastole. The murmur is the result of turbulent blood flow across the stenotic valve, which occurs during the filling of the left ventricle.

54. **B.** Aortic regurgitation results in the back-flow of blood across the valve into the left ventricle during diastole. This murmur is best heard at the third and fourth intercostal space at the *left* sternal border when it is due to aortic *valve* disease, and at the *right* sternal border when it is due to aortic *root* disease (*Right = Root*). In severe cases, a second diastolic murmur can be heard in the area of the left lower sternal border. This murmur, known as the Austin-Flint murmur, is the result of the regurgitant stream of blood striking the mitral leaflets and making a "relative" mitral stenosis.

55. **E.** Similar to mitral stenosis, tricuspid stenosis results in turbulent blood flow across the valve during filling of the right ventricle (diastole). This murmur, however, is best heard in the area of the tricuspid valve (left lower sternal border).

56. **A.** AS results in turbulence of blood flow across the valve during ejection of the blood from the left ventricle (systole). It is best heard in the right upper sternal border area and often radiates into the carotids.

57. **D.** The murmur of mitral regurgitation, which is best heard in the apical area, results from retrograde blood flow across the insufficient valve into the left atrium during systole.

58. **F.** Tricuspid regurgitation is similar to mitral regurgitation, in that the murmur is the result of retrograde blood flow across the valve during systole. It can be distinguished from mitral regurgitation because as a general rule right-sided murmurs increase in intensity with inspiration. This is because blood is "sucked" into the right atrium with the negative intrathoracic pressure that occurs during inspiration and increases the volume of blood that travels across the stenotic or regurgitant valve. Tricuspid regurgitation is also heard best in the area of the tricuspid valve (along the left lower sternal border) as opposed to the apical area where mitral regurgitation is best heard.

G. Although a PDA can result in a murmur along the left sternal border, it is usually closer to the clavicular area and is a continuous "machine gun" type of murmur (i.e., it is heard throughout systole and diastole).

H. The murmur of coarctation of the aorta sounds similar to AS, but it is often heard in the upper back area. Checking the peripheral pulses also helps distinguish between AS and coarctation of the aorta. In coarctation of the aorta, the pulses in the lower extremities are diminished when compared with the pulses in the upper extremities. AS should not result in a discrepancy in the peripheral pulses.

59. | **E.** A CT scan of the chest is the test of choice to evaluate for a possible thoracic dissection. It is the most rapid and precise test that is readily available. The classic finding of a dissection on CT is widening of the aorta with extravasation of blood into the wall of the aorta causing the "double barrel" sign.

A. The ECG may show evidence of ischemia if the coronary arteries are involved, but otherwise is not useful in the diagnosis of thoracic aortic dissection.

B. Chest X-ray may show widening of the mediastinum, which should raise concern for dissection, but it does not confirm the diagnosis or identify the exact portion of the aorta that is involved. It also cannot be used to estimate the size of the dissection.

C. TEE will give a better assessment of the descending portion of the aorta, and is also a good way to assess the ascending aorta, next to the aortic valve. However, TEE is not as readily available as a CT scan. In addition, if there is any concern or evidence of an acute myocardial infarction, then a TEE is contraindicated. However, if the patient is in the ICU and is too unstable to go to CT scan, an emergent TEE is a good option to diagnose a dissection of the aorta.

D. TTE is a relatively rapid, noninvasive way of assessing cardiac function and valvular abnormalities. However, the aortic root and ascending aorta are not always well visualized on echocardiogram. In addition, the descending aorta is difficult to thoroughly assess with the transthoracic approach, thereby increasing your chances of missing the diagnosis.

60. | **B.** This patient's condition is a medical emergency and the first step in the treatment of the dissection is to rapidly decrease his blood pressure. This is best accomplished by using IV medications such as nitroprusside and β-blockers. Nitroprusside should be used with a β-blocker, not alone. If nitroprusside is used alone, the arterial vasodilatory properties will cause a reflex tachycardia that can worsen "shearing forces" in the dissection. Therefore, it is important to use arterial vasodilators at the same time as β-blockers to avoid this phenomenon.

A. Transfusing platelets and fresh-frozen plasma may be necessary during his operative procedure or postoperatively; however, it will do nothing acutely to stop the advancement of his dissection.

C. Dissections of the ascending aorta almost always require surgical intervention, so a cardiothoracic surgery consult should be obtained expeditiously. However, attempts at reduction in blood pressure should be initiated while you are awaiting the arrival of the surgical team.

D. Observing the patient with serial echocardiograms is not acceptable management. This patient has a medical emergency requiring prompt and rapid treatment (including surgical intervention). Simply observing this patient is putting him at significant risk of death.

E. Although blood pressure may be treated with oral ACE-inhibitors, this is not appropriate given the longer onset of action of the oral medications and the need for immediate reduction of blood pressure.

61. **B.** Although lung cancer is second to breast cancer in incidence for women in the United States, it is the most common cause of cancer *death*. Lung cancer accounts for 12% of cancers in this population, but accounts for 25% of cancer deaths.

A. Colorectal cancer accounts for 11% of cancer incidence in this population and 11% of cancer deaths. This makes it the third most common cancer and the third leading cause of cancer death for women in the United States.

C. Breast cancer has the highest incidence of cancers among women in the United States, accounting for 30% of cancers. However, it falls behind lung cancer as a cause of cancer death at 15%.

D. Leukemia accounts for only 4% of cancer deaths among women in the United States. Leukemia makes up less than 2% of cancer types for this population.

E. Ovarian cancer accounts for 4% of cancers among women in the United States, making it the fifth most common cancer in women. Additionally, it is the fifth leading cause of cancer death in this population, accounting for 5% of all cancer deaths.

62. **C.** When evaluating breast masses, the clinical suspicion for cancer and the age of the patient help to guide the work-up. Mammograms are less diagnostic in premenopausal women because of the generally higher density of the breast tissue. Therefore, a palpable mass in a 70-year-old woman should trigger a mammogram evaluation. A palpable mass in a woman who is age 35 or younger is better evaluated by an initial ultrasound to determine whether the mass is cystic or solid. *It is important to remember that a patient with a persistent palpable breast mass who has a normal mammogram still requires further work-up.*

A. Ultrasound can determine whether the lesion is a simple cyst or if it has septations and/or solid components. An excisional biopsy may be indicated *after* the ultrasound, if the ultrasound determines that the lesion is not a simple cyst.

B. See explanation for C.

D. Mastectomy should be undertaken only after a tissue diagnosis of cancer is obtained and treatment options are discussed with the patient.

E. Occasionally, it may be reasonable in a woman who is considered very low risk for cancer to be observed through one menstrual cycle to determine if the mass lesion goes away with normal hormone fluctuations. However, this patient had observed the lesion through three menstrual cycles without any change in the lesion, and therefore it warrants further evaluation.

63. **D.** A younger age at menarche is a known risk factor for breast cancer. The longer time of menses increases exposure to hormones, thereby increasing risk of breast cancer. The average age of menarche in the United States is 12.2 years, so this patient has undergone menarche relatively early at age 10.

A. A personal history of breast cancer increases the risk of new or recurrent cancer in either breast. Our patient did not have a personal history of breast cancer.

B. The number of first-degree relatives with breast cancer increases the risk. First-degree relatives include mother, sisters, and daughters. One first-degree relative affected increases the risk by almost two-fold. However, this patient had an aunt with breast cancer.

C. Whites have the highest rate of breast cancer after age 40. Black women have the second-highest rate, but the highest mortality. Hispanic women have the third-highest rate of breast cancer.

E. Older age at first live birth increases the risk of breast cancer. Women who give birth at age 35 or more have 1.5 times the risk of breast cancer than those who give birth before age 25.

64. | **D.** This patient meets the Amsterdam Criteria for diagnosis of HNPCC (also known as Lynch syndrome). It is inherited in an autosomal dominant pattern. The Amsterdam Criteria are: three or more relatives with colorectal cancer, one affected relative is a first-degree relative, two generations of family with colorectal cancer, and one case is diagnosed in a family member younger than fifty years of age. Although it is often difficult to distinguish HNPCC from FAP, the findings on colonoscopy should rule out FAP in this case (see explanation for A).

A. FAP typically presents in the second to third decade of life. FAP is caused by a mutation in the adenomatous polyposis coli (APC) gene and is transmitted in an autosomal dominant manner. Multiple polyps, typically 500 to 2500 polyps "carpeting" the mucosal surface, can be found on colonoscopy. There is a tremendous risk that these polyps will transform into adenocarcinoma of the colon over time.

B. BRCA-1 mutation is associated with breast cancer, ovarian cancer, and prostate cancer.

C. Gardner's syndrome is a subset of familial APC. In addition to the colonic polyps, patients also have soft tissue and bony tumors and ampullary cancers.

E. Peutz-Jeghers syndrome is a rare autosomal dominant syndrome characterized by multiple hamartomatous polyps scattered throughout the gastrointestinal tract. Patients have small macular "freckle" appearing areas of pigmentation on the oral mucosa, lips, face, and palmar surface of the hands. Although the hamartomatous polyps carry no risk of malignancy, the patients are at risk of pancreatic, lung, breast, ovarian, and uterine cancers.

65. | **B.** Screening recommendations for family members include a colonoscopy at age 20 to 25 years OR 10 years younger than the age of diagnosis for the youngest person in the family, whichever comes first. This should be repeated every 1 to 2 years because of the rapid progression of malignancy in these patients, even if the first colonoscopy is normal.

A. Fecal occult blood testing, a screening test used in the general population, is not adequate in this patient population.

C. Female family members are at increased risk for endometrial and ovarian cancer. Annual screening for these malignancies should begin at age 25. Screening includes pelvic examination with endometrial aspirate or transvaginal ultrasound.

D. Colonoscopy should be repeated more frequently than is recommended for the general population. Current recommendations are to repeat the exam every 1 to 2 years.

E. Flexible sigmoidoscopy is not adequate to screen for colon cancer in this patient population. The entire colon must be examined.

66. **C.** This patient has small cell carcinoma (also called "oat cell" carcinoma) of the lung. The cancer is highly malignant and is in the family of small, round, blue (basophilic-staining) tumors of neuroendocrine origin. Small cell carcinomas often produce paraneoplastic syndromes because of their production of ectopic hormones such as ACTH (resulting in Cushing's syndrome). Other, less well-known paraneoplastic syndromes include subacute cortical cerebellar degeneration, which presents as vertigo, dysarthria, diplopia, and nystagmus. It is thought to be due to antibody-mediated destruction of the cerebellar Purkinje cells and their axons.

A. The prognosis for small cell carcinoma is poor, both with and without treatment. Without treatment, life expectancy is 2 to 4 months. Staging is simple: Limited-stage disease (30% of patients) means that the disease is confined to one hemithorax and its regional lymph nodes. Extensive-stage disease is that which is not confined to the above "limits."

B. Treatment with chemotherapy with or without radiation can prolong the duration and quality of life for those with small cell lung cancer, but overall the prognosis is not very good. There is no role for surgery in the treatment of small cell lung cancer.

D. Small cell lung cancer is highly related to smoking. Only 1% of patients with the disease are nonsmokers.

E. The tumor arises from neuroendocrine cells of the lining of bronchial epithelium.

67. **B.** Burkitt's lymphoma is a type of non-Hodgkin's lymphoma. Patients with this type of lymphoma can present with a rapidly enlarging mass on the head or neck. African Burkitt's lymphoma cells express the Epstein-Barr virus receptor and have the EBV virus genome in the tumor cells.

68. **C.** *H. pylori* infection has a known association with gastric MALT lymphoma. MALT lymphoma can progress to large B-cell lymphoma.

69. **A.** Adult T-cell lymphoma is associated with HTLV-1 infection. Adult T-cell lymphoma presents with diffuse adenopathy, hepatosplenomegaly, cutaneous lesions, hypercalcemia, lytic bone lesions, and interstitial pulmonary infiltrates. The WBC count is high, and peripheral smear shows highly convoluted, abnormal nuclei.

D. CMV is not associated with a lymphoma.

E. HHV-8 has been linked to Kaposi's sarcoma, but not to lymphoma.

70. **B.** This man is presenting with painless jaundice, anorexia, and weight loss over a time period of several weeks. He has a significant smoking history that is a risk factor for pancreatic cancer. Obstruction of the biliary tree by the mass leads to jaundice. Obstruction of the duodenum leads to nausea and vomiting. Often patients will also have dull epigastric and back pain which they may describe as "gnawing" or "boring" in quality.

A. Cholecystitis is caused by obstruction of the cystic duct by a gallstone. This patient does not present with a history of right upper quadrant pain, fever, or vomiting after meals. There is no tenderness to palpation over the right upper quadrant on exam, and his WBC count is normal. These findings go against a diagnosis of cholecystitis. In addition, cholecystitis by itself should not cause jaundice, unless a stone is obstructing the bile duct; in this case, the more likely diagnosis is ascending cholangitis.

C. The classic presentation for ascending cholangitis is fever, jaundice, and right upper quadrant pain. Cholangitis is an infection proximal to obstruction of the common bile duct.

D. Gilbert's syndrome is a mild, persistent, unconjugated (indirect) hyperbilirubinemia caused by a decrease in glucuronosyltransferase activity. This is the enzyme that conjugates bilirubin from the indirect portion to the direct portion. It is a common syndrome, thought to be present in 3% to 10% of the general population. The total bilirubin usually runs from 1.5 to 3.0 mg/dL, and rarely exceeds 5.0 mg/dL, and it will be mostly indirect. A feature of Gilbert's that can be diagnostically useful is that the indirect bilirubin increases after fasting. Our patient does not display any of these features.

E. Autoimmune hemolytic anemia would not cause a direct hyperbilirubinemia as in our patient. The hemoglobin is usually low and the mean corpuscular volume (MCV) is usually elevated because of the larger size of the reticulocytes that are being pumped out of the bone marrow to make up for the decreased life span of the hemolyzed red cells.

71. **E.** One of the symptoms of multiple myeloma is bone pain. Radiographs of the bones affected will show "punched out" lesions due to activation of osteoclasts by the cytokines released by the malignant cells. Multiple myeloma occurs as a result of a monoclonal malignant proliferation of plasma cells. The malignant plasma cells secrete immunoglobulins, which are reflected in the elevated serum total protein, and should make you think of the diagnosis. Additional findings of this disease include anemia, hypercalcemia, and renal failure. Anemia occurs secondary to the decreased RBC production by the bone marrow. Bone pain, lytic lesions, and hypercalcemia are due to increased osteoclastic activity. Renal failure occurs as a result of the toxic effects of the light chains on the renal tubules. Recurrent infections are due to hypogammaglobulinemia of all other immunoglobulins except the monoclonal (M) chain. Diagnosis can be made by serum protein electrophoresis (SPEP) or urine protein electrophoresis (UPEP). SPEP detects the M component and UPEP detects a light chain predominance.

A. Acute lymphocytic leukemia typically presents in children, but can occur in adults. Patients present with fatigue and bone pain. Hepatosplenomegaly, lymphadenopathy, and an anterior mediastinal mass are often present. Punched-out lesions and hypercalcemia are not present.

B. MGUS occurs when there is only an elevation of total serum protein with predominance of M component. The other findings that are seen with multiple myeloma, including renal failure, anemia, punched-out bone lesions, and hypercalcemia, are not present with MGUS. Approximately 25% of patients with MGUS progress to multiple myeloma.

C. Waldenström's macroglobulinemia is a low-grade proliferation of plasmacytoid lymphocyte cells that secrete IgM. There are no bone lesions. Patients can have symptoms related to hyperviscosity.

D. Chronic myelogenous leukemia presents in the chronic phase with fevers, night sweats, fatigue, and splenomegaly. They do not have bone lesions.

72. | **B.** This presentation is consistent with Hodgkin's lymphoma. There is a bimodal distribution of disease at ages 15 to 35 and again over 50. Patients usually present with lymphadenopathy including mediastinal adenopathy. "B" symptoms include fever, night sweats, and weight loss. When Reed-Sternberg cells are found on lymph node biopsy, the diagnosis of Hodgkin's disease can be made with certainty. The malignant cells are frequently binucleate and more closely resemble macrophages than lymphocytes.

A. CMV is a virus in the herpes family. It has a number of clinical presentations including neonatal infection, primary infection in late childhood or adulthood (which resembles a mononucleosis-type illness), and infection of immunocompromised patients. Cytomegalic cells are infected epithelial cells that are two to four times the size of the surrounding cells. They have an 8- to 10-μm intranuclear inclusion that is eccentrically placed and surrounded by a clear halo that looks like an "owl's eye." This patient does not have hepatosplenomegaly, which is common with primary CMV in an adult. Also, the lymph node biopsy reveals a Reed-Sternberg cell.

C. Non-Hodgkin's lymphoma typically presents with painless lymphadenopathy and may also have "B" symptoms. Reed-Sternberg cells are diagnostic for Hodgkin's lymphoma, however, not non-Hodgkin's lymphoma.

D. Scrofula (or tuberculous lymphadenitis) is in the differential of a firm lymph node often in the cervical region. Patients may or may not have evidence of prior tuberculosis on chest X-ray. The biopsy should show acid-fast bacillus (AFB) organisms, however, not Reed-Sternberg cells.

E. Sarcoidosis may manifest with mediastinal adenopathy and the malaise and dyspnea that our patient feels. However, the biopsy of the nodes would reveal noncaseating granulomas consistent with sarcoidosis.

73. | **D.** Simple measures such as elevation of the head of the bed, providing oxygen, and gentle diuresis can improve the patient's symptoms while a diagnosis is pursued.

A. Lung cancer is the leading cause of SVC syndrome. Lymphoma is the second leading cause. Other causes include infection and clot formation from catheters or pacer wires.

B. Glucocorticoids and acute airway management should be the first step in management of a patient with tracheal obstruction due to SVC syndrome. Radiation may be used later in treatment if appropriate for diagnosis.

C. The most common physical finding is cervical venous distension. Other physical findings include facial edema, facial plethora, cyanosis, and conjunctival edema.

E. Radiation can affect prognosis if the underlying tumor is radiation responsive.

74. | **E.** Sensitivity and specificity are two statistical formulas that are used to help evaluate clinical tests. The sensitivity is the ratio of patients *with* a disease who have a positive test divided by all the patients with the disease. A test with high sensitivity will result in very few patients with false-negative results. In other words, it will not miss many patients who have the disease. Therefore, if a test with high sensitivity is negative, the patient most likely does not have the disease, making it a good test for "ruling out" the disease. Specificity is the ratio of all the patients *without* a disease who have a negative test result divided by all the patients who do not have the disease. A test with high specificity will have very few false positives. Therefore, if you use a test with high specificity to screen for a disease, a patient with a positive result most likely has the disease, making it a good test to "rule in" the disease. To calculate the sensitivity and specificity of a particular test, you need to know the total number of people tested, the prevalence of the disease, and the results of the test. In our example, 1000 people were tested and the disease prevalence was high (20%). Table 74 is an example of a "two by two table" that illustrates this concept applied to our results. Of the 1000 patients tested, 200 actually have the disease that we are screening for (20%) and 800 do not. Of the 200 that do have the disease, 180 have a positive test result, making the sensitivity 90%. The specificity of this test would then be 80%.

■ TABLE 74	Two by Two Table	
	Patients *with* the disease	Patients *without* the disease
+ test results	180 (True Positive)	160 (False Positive)
− test results	20 (False Negative)	640 (True Negative)
Sensitivity = True Positives/(True Positives + False Negatives)		
Specificity = True Negatives/(True Negatives + False Positives)		

A, B, C, D. See explanation for E.

75. **A.** The term "liver function tests" can be somewhat misleading, so one must be careful when analyzing them. The tests that are often included in the hepatic function panel include the AST, ALT, bilirubin, alkaline phosphatase, albumin, and total protein. Of these tests, the albumin is the only test that truly reflects the synthetic function of the liver (as does the PT, which is not included above). The levels of AST, ALT, alkaline phosphatase, and bilirubin do not necessarily correlate with the functional status of the liver. In other words, the AST (or other labs listed above) can be elevated, but the function of the liver may not be compromised. These tests give the clinician insight into the type of process occurring when these laboratory values are abnormal. Typically, these abnormalities can be categorized as either "obstructive" or "hepatocellular injury." With hepatocellular injury (without obstruction), one would expect to see increased AST and ALT levels, because these are dumped into the bloodstream from the injured cells. However, you would not expect to see significant increase in the bilirubin or alkaline phosphatase levels. In an obstructive process, such as cholelithiasis or choledocholithiasis, the biliary tree is unable to drain normally. As biliary fluid accumulates behind the obstruction, one would expect to see increases in the bilirubin and alkaline phosphatase levels. When this blockage occurs, some mild hepatocellular injury can be revealed by an increase in the AST and ALT levels, but not to the same extent as with other processes. Processes which cause hepatocellular injury can have varying degrees of injury. For example, in alcohol-induced hepatitis, one typically sees an increase in the AST and ALT into the low hundreds range. Classically, AST to ALT is at a ratio of 2:1 to 3:1. However, in viral hepatitis (most commonly type A or B), one sees a significantly higher degree of cellular injury with higher transaminase values (in the thousands). There are only a handful of conditions that can cause a person's AST and ALT to reach the thousands. Other conditions include viral hepatitis, acetaminophen (or other drug) toxicity, ischemia (shock liver), and sometimes autoimmune disease.

B. Cholelithiasis would show more of an obstructive picture. One would expect to see the bilirubin and alkaline phosphatase higher, with only mild increases in AST and ALT.

C. See explanation for A.

D. Hemochromatosis is an infiltrative disease in which excess iron is deposited into the tissue of the liver. The liver function tests can be normal or show mild evidence of hepatocellular injury, but should not reveal this presentation or degree of injury.

E. Changes due to hepatocellular carcinoma should give a picture of hepatocellular injury. However, if the tumor is encroaching on or compressing an intrahepatic duct or the biliary tree, an obstructive picture may also be present. Hepatocellular carcinoma is most commonly seen in patients who are already cirrhotic, usually from chronic viral hepatitis.

76. **E.** As in the explanation to question 75, there are only a few conditions that can cause ALT and AST levels to reach into the thousands: viral hepatitis, acetaminophen toxicity, liver ischemia, and sometimes autoimmune disease. In this scenario it would be advisable to check an acute hepatitis panel and an acetaminophen level (this was not a choice, however).

A. Abdominal ultrasound is the recommended radiologic study to evaluate for cholelithiasis, but it is not necessarily useful in the diagnosis of viral hepatitis.

B. It would be reasonable to check an ethanol level in a patient if you felt the liver injury pattern was consistent with alcoholic hepatitis. However, alcohol should not increase transaminases to these levels, and should give an AST : ALT ratio of 2:1 to 3:1.

C. Percutaneous liver biopsy would be indicated if there were concern for hepatocellular carcinoma or if the underlying diagnosis was not clear. However, in this case, the changes in the liver function tests would not be typically seen in a patient with hepatocellular carcinoma.

D. Percentage of transferrin saturated with iron (also known as % sat) would be useful in helping assess a patient for hemochromatosis, but this disease would not result in the degree of transaminase elevation seen in this patient.

77. **C.** This patient has a new lesion present in his lung and has risk factors for cancer (age and smoking). Therefore, a tissue specimen should be obtained to make certain this is not cancer. If the lesion had been present on a previous chest X-ray and had not changed for 2 years, then one could conceivably follow it clinically with follow-up chest X-rays. However, we do not have the luxury of previous chest X-rays on this patient. To wait and follow this lesion may allow a possibly malignant tumor to grow and metastasize. The location of the lesion is helpful in determining the best approach to obtaining a biopsy. Central lesions are usually accessible by bronchoscopy with biopsy. However, peripheral lesions, such as the one in our patient, are not as easily accessible with the bronchoscope, so CT-guided needle biopsy is the method of choice.

A, B. New or suspicious pulmonary lesions should be evaluated promptly to exclude the presence of a malignant lesion. Having him follow up in 3 or 6 months for a repeat chest X-ray is not an acceptable way of managing this patient.

D. See explanation for C.

E. The presence of an upper lobe lesion should raise your concern about the possibility of mycobacterial disease (e.g., tuberculosis). Although there is a small possibility this could be the cause of this patient's lesion, it is unlikely. Placing a PPD skin test is not a bad idea in this clinical setting, but it is not the most appropriate next step in working up this patient.

78. | **B.** This patient is at high risk for the development of DVT and subsequent PE and should therefore be started on prophylactic therapy. There are several possible treatments that can prevent VTE. These include subcutaneous administration of unfractionated heparin at 5000 U every 8 to 12 hours or low-molecular weight heparins on a reduced dosing schedule (e.g., enoxaparin 40 U subcutaneously once a day).

A. See explanation for B.

C, E. If the patient has a risk of bleeding that would make you want to avoid such anticoagulation medications as low-dose heparin, you may use sequential compression devices on the lower extremities. However, the graduated compression stockings and sequential compression devices are not appropriate to use alone in patients who are at high risk of DVT. Only moderate- to low-risk patients, or patients at high risk of significant bleeding, should be given SCDs alone.

D. Full-dose anticoagulation with IV heparin or full-dose anticoagulation with low molecular weight heparin is indicated for the treatment of VTE, but not prevention of VTE, as in this patient.

79. | **D.** Patients who are admitted to the hospital have altered physiologic and metabolic processes due to their illnesses. Some of these patients have a higher risk of stress-related gastric ulcers and subsequent upper GI bleeding events. Hospital patients who should be placed on stress ulcer prophylaxis are those who are intubated, are coagulopathic (i.e., at risk for bleeding), or have prior histories of upper GI bleeding. The man described in example D has two of the three risk factors and is therefore at the highest risk.

A, B, C, E. See explanation for D.

80. | **C.** The four most common causes of chronic cough include asthma, gastroesophageal reflux, postnasal drip, and allergies. Of these, her history is most suggestive of reflux-type symptoms, because the cough is worse with being supine and she has frequent heartburn.

A, B, D. She does not have classic symptoms of cough secondary to asthma (wheezing, worse at night, identifiable triggers) or postnasal drip (worse in the morning, nasal congestion, etc.).

E. Although bronchogenic carcinoma can cause a persistent cough, it is usually seen in patients with a history of tobacco abuse, which she denies. It is also usually associated with other symptoms such as weight loss and hemoptysis, neither of which she reports.

81. **C.** When assessing a patient with dysphagia, it is helpful to assess whether their symptoms are caused only by solids or if they also occur when drinking liquids. This helps to distinguish between a motility disorder and an underlying obstructive lesion. With a motility disorder, the patient should have symptoms with both solids and liquids. With an obstructive lesion in the esophagus (e.g., a tumor), you would expect solids to stick but liquids to pass without difficulty. Determining whether symptoms are intermittent or progressive also helps the diagnosis. Problems such as diffuse esophageal spasm and esophageal rings are usually intermittent, whereas achalasia and tumors are progressive. This patient reports progressive dysphagia with solids only, which is concerning for possible malignancy. The two main types of esophageal cancer are adenocarcinoma and squamous cell carcinoma. Patients at increased risk for adenocarcinoma are those with long-standing untreated gastroesophageal reflux and Barrett's esophagus. Adenocarcinoma usually affects the distal portion of the esophagus near the gastroesophageal junction. Squamous cell carcinoma typically affects the midportion of the esophagus and is more prevalent in patients who abuse tobacco and alcohol. Therefore, given this patient's history, he is at risk of esophageal adenocarcinoma. The appropriate diagnostic test is an EGD with biopsy.

A. Achalasia typically presents with progressive dysphagia with solids and liquids, which this patient does not report. An upper GI can be done to evaluate for achalasia, but this is not the most likely diagnosis.

B, D, E. See explanation for C.

82. **E.** This patient likely has a breast cyst, given the physical exam findings of smoothness, fluctuance, and mild tenderness. The timing of the breast mass with her period is also suggestive of a breast cyst. Fibrocystic disease is the most common cause of a breast mass in premenopausal women.

A. Breast adenocarcinoma on physical exam is often firm, irregular, nontender, and fixed.

B. Fibrous adenomas are common in this age group but tend to persist throughout several menstrual cycles.

C. Breast abscesses are seen in lactating women, and the bacterial etiology is usually *Staphylococcus aureus* or *Streptococcus*. This patient is not lactating and does not give any history of fevers or chills, so a breast abscess is less likely.

D. Fat necrosis occurs with trauma and presents as a firm, tender mass.

83. **B.** Since this mass has not disappeared, it is likely that it is a fibroadenoma. The next step in evaluation of the mass is to perform an ultrasound. Doctors who are trained in the procedure of fine needle aspiration will sometimes put a needle in the part of the breast that is suspicious for a cyst to see if it is possible to aspirate fluid before ordering the ultrasound. If the fluid that is aspirated is clear and the lump goes away, then it is reasonable to follow the patient to see if the fluid reaccumulates. If the lump returns, then it must be evaluated further with ultrasound. If the aspirated fluid is bloody, it must be sent for cytology, and further evaluation with ultrasound should be done. If the mass on ultrasound appears solid, then the patient *must* have a tissue diagnosis made, either by excisional biopsy, fine needle, or core biopsy.

A. BRCA-1 and BRCA-2 gene mutations are associated with malignant disease. There are many questions that must be asked when deciding to test for such genes, such as, "What is the sensitivity and specificity of the test?" and "Is there a proven intervention available?" Testing for BRCA-1 and -2 is not recommended for people at average risk for breast cancer because of the incidence of false positives in that population. It is appropriate for a patient with a strong family history of breast cancer to consider gene testing; however, it is not currently recommended to test for the gene in other patients except in research protocols. Given our patient's history, physical exam, and family history, she would not be a candidate for gene testing.

C. A mammogram is not as sensitive or specific in a woman younger than age 35 as it is in older women, because of the relatively higher density of premenopausal breast tissue. It is recommended that the evaluation of a palpable lump in a woman who is 35 or younger be initiated with an ultrasound as opposed to a mammogram. In a woman older than 35, it is reasonable to start the evaluation of a lump with a mammogram. However, if the mammogram is normal, further imaging needs to be done and, eventually, perhaps a biopsy.

D. See explanation for B.

E. It would be negligent to wait on this patient's breast mass, especially because it did not disappear after her period.

84. **B.** Any woman who presents with secondary amenorrhea (meaning that she has had periods in the past that have now ceased) needs evaluation for possible pregnancy as the cause. Even though this patient states that she could not be pregnant because of her use of condoms with her boyfriend, you need to check a pregnancy test. If she is not pregnant, then she is probably having intermittent anovulatory cycles that account for her irregular periods. Anovulatory cycles are common in adolescents in the first 2 to 3 years after menarche secondary to an immature hypothalamic-pituitary-ovarian axis.

A. Oral contraceptive pills have many uses; they are used for contraception, in patients with dysfunctional uterine bleeding to decrease the amount of endometrium shed, and in patients with polycystic ovarian syndrome. They can also be used to regulate the cycles of women with irregular cycles, such as this patient. An oral contraceptive pill may be used in her future, but is not the next step in her evaluation.

C. Basal body temperatures are often used in the fertility process to determ a woman is ovulating, noted by a rise in temperature after ovulation secondary increased progesterone. It is not something to recommend to our patient at this point.

D. A TSH could be measured if there were a concern that hypothyroidism was caus- ing her irregular cycles. Hypothyroidism, if it effects the menstrual cycle, usually manifests as heavy flow, or menorrhagia.

E. Endometrial biopsy is indicated in all women over the age of 35 with abnormal uterine bleeding to rule out cancer or premalignant lesions. This does not apply to our patient.

85. **D.** Acute angle-closure glaucoma usually presents with a deep aching pain, nausea, and vomiting. Other clues to the diagnosis include a mid-dilated fixed pupil that is unresponsive to light and clouding of the cornea. It is considered an emergency and needs to be evaluated right away by measuring the intraocular pressures and consulting an ophthalmologist.

A. Viral conjunctivitis is usually preceded by an upper respiratory infection and is usually bilateral. Often, there is discharge. There is no effect on vision or pupillary response to light.

B. Keratitis results in inflammation of the corneal limbus and may result in ulceration of the cornea. It may be caused by bacteria, fungi, or viruses and can present with irritation, photophobia, and tearing. When it is due to herpes simplex, which is the most common cause of keratitis in the United States, it is minimally painful, which can be very helpful diagnostically. If the center of the cornea is affected, there may be reduction in vision.

C. Allergic conjunctivitis is usually associated with itchy, watery eyes and other atopic symptoms such as clear rhinorrhea and sneezing. It is usually bilateral and nonpainful, and the pupils react normally. There is no vision loss.

E. Corneal abrasions usually present as excruciating eye pain with the sensation of a foreign body present in the eye. The patient will often give you a history that "something got in my eye" and the initial foreign body sensation progressed to severe pain. Photophobia is the result of painful contraction of the hyperemic iris. Often, the use of anesthetic drops can help in the examination of the eye. The pupil should be normally reactive.

86. **C.** According to the guidelines of the American Society for Colposcopy and Cervical Pathology (ASCCP) that were based on the ALTS trial (Atypical Squa- mous Cells of Undetermined Significance/Low-Grade Squamous Intraepithe- lial Lesions Triage study), patients who present with ASCUS on Pap should undergo HPV serotyping to check whether they are at high or low risk for ma- lignancy. If the serotype is low risk, then it is reasonable to put them back into the normal cervical cancer screening group, and repeat the Pap smear in 1 year. If the serotype is high risk, then the next step would be colposcopy with biopsy, and possible cryotherapy if needed.

ot continue to keep a patient in the normal screening population cat-
hey have had an abnormal Pap smear. You cannot wait for a year to
e abnormal Pap.

xplanation for C.

---

87. **D.** Colon cancer is the second leading cause of cancer death in the United States. Once someone has a positive fecal occult blood test, the next step is to perform a colonoscopy to evaluate for cancer.

A. Single contrast barium enemas are used in older patients or patients who are unable to tolerate the air injected in a double contrast enema. It is not as sensitive as colonoscopy to look for polyps or small cancers and is not recommended.

B. Anoscopy can be done to look for bleeding of the hemorrhoids, but the evaluation should *not* stop there. A patient with guaiac-positive stool needs to have evaluation of the *entire* colon to look for cancerous or precancerous lesions.

C. Flexible sigmoidoscopy is not recommended, because the patient needs to have the entire colon examined.

E. A CT scan of the abdomen and pelvis can aid in looking for metastatic lesions, but does not give direct visualization of the mucosal surface of the colon, and small polyps or cancers can be missed.

---

88. **C.** The combination OCP is a good choice for birth control for women who are able to take a pill consistently every day. Other advantages include decreased menstrual flow and dysmenorrheic symptoms, improvement of acne with certain formulations, and decreased risk of ovarian cancer over time. It is not a good choice for birth control for women who are not able to take pills consistently. It also does not protect against STDs, including those with no cure such as herpes, HPV, or HIV.

---

89. **B.** Injectable progesterone in a depo form (Depo-Provera) is a birth control option for women who do not want to have to take a pill every day. It is given every 3 months in an intramuscular injection. Side effects include irregular bleeding and eventual amenorrhea in most women, acne, and minimal weight gain. Like OCPs, it does not protect against STDs.

---

90. **A.** Progesterone-containing IUDs are birth-control options for women who do not want to take a pill every day and do not want intramuscular injections. It is an object that must be inserted by a gynecologist, and there is a low possibility of mechanical complications such as uterine perforation. Patients who are in monogamous relationships are better candidates for the device, because there is an increased risk of PID in patients with IUDs who are having sex with multiple partners.

91. **D.** Condoms and diaphragms are forms of barrier contraception. They have a better chance of preventing pregnancy when they are used in combination with a spermicide-containing product. Condoms can help to prevent the spread of HIV and other STDs, but they are not perfect and do not protect well against HPV, which is the virus that causes cervical cancer.

92. **B.** This patient has bacterial vaginosis caused by *Gardnerella vaginalis*. Risk factors for vaginosis include early age of onset of intercourse, multiple sex partners, cigarette smoking, and douching. Other diagnostic criteria include a pH >4.5 and a positive whiff test (fishy odor upon application of KOH to vaginal discharge samples). The cells on the wet mount fit the description of "clue cells," which are epithelial cells coated with the *G. vaginalis* bacteria.

A. This patient's urinalysis is normal, so urinary tract infection is unlikely.

C. Patients with trichomoniasis often present with dysuria, pruritus, and discharge, and may have punctate "strawberry spot" lesions on the cervix. Patients may also have intense pruritus and a frothy, watery, greenish-gray discharge.

D. *Chlamydia*, like trichomoniasis, is sexually transmitted and presents with vaginal discharge, burning, and itching. It can also be asymptomatic. It is diagnosed by antigen detection of cervical swab specimens, by genetic probe methods of cervical swabs, or most recently by nucleic acid amplification techniques to detect the organism in urine specimens. The nucleic acid amplification techniques are extremely sensitive for *Chlamydia* detection, are convenient because they don't require a pelvic exam, and can be done on urine specimens, which are less invasive.

E. Vaginal candidiasis presents with dysuria, irritation, dyspareunia, and a thick, white clumpy discharge. The yeasts (spores and/or pseudohyphae) are seen on KOH wet mount.

93. **C.** Metronidazole is first-line treatment for patients with bacterial vaginosis. It is also used in the treatment of trichomoniasis.

A, B. Trimethoprim-sulfamethoxazole and ciprofloxacin are used for treatment of the uncomplicated urinary tract infection.

D. Diflucan, in a one-time dose, is used for treatment of candidiasis. Other topical antifungal agents can be used as well.

E. Ceftriaxone is used to treat *Neisseria gonorrhoeae* infection.

94. **D.** The definitive criteria for the diagnosis of diabetes include a fasting glucose >126, a random glucose >200 with symptoms of polyuria and polydipsia, or a 2-hour postprandial glucose greater than 200. HgbA1C measurements are not considered diagnostic criteria for diabetes.

E. Glucose on urine dip can be present from hyperglycemia or an inability of the kidneys to reabsorb glucose, as seen in Fanconi's syndrome.

A, B, C. See explanation for D.

95. **C.** Urge incontinence is caused by an overactive urinary bladder detrusor muscle. The patient describes an intense, sudden urge to urinate that may be difficult to control. Patients may avoid social situations because of the fear of accidents. Often, the etiology of detrusor muscle spasm is idiopathic, but bacterial cystitis must be ruled out.

D. Stress incontinence is seen in patients with weak pelvic floor muscles and presents with incontinence during coughing, sneezing, or laughing. These actions cause increased intra-abdominal pressure, which allows the hypermobile urethra to move and allows urine to leak. Ten percent of patients may have intrinsic sphincter deficiency as a cause of their stress incontinence. Risk factors for stress incontinence include aging, estrogen deficiency, a prior traumatic vaginal delivery, or pelvic surgery. Stress incontinence is the most common cause of urinary incontinence in younger women, and the second most common cause of urinary incontinence in older women.

E. Overflow incontinence is secondary to weakened detrusor activity and/or bladder outlet obstruction. Postvoid residual is usually elevated in overflow incontinence (>100 mL) and the stream is often hesitant.

A, B. See explanations for C, D, and E.

96. **D.** This patient has the classic presentation of community-acquired pneumonia (CAP) caused by *Streptococcus pneumoniae*, which includes abrupt onset of high fevers with rigors, productive cough with rust-colored sputum, pleuritic chest pain, and a lobar consolidation on chest X-ray. Although any of the organisms listed above may cause pneumonia, they typically have a different natural history and affect different hosts.

A. *M. pneumoniae* is one of the organisms responsible for causing an "atypical" form of CAP. Patients with *M. pneumoniae* generally have a more indolent course with low-grade fevers and cough and usually do not appear so abruptly ill. On chest X-ray, they can have focal consolidative changes, but chest X-rays can range from normal to those with patchy bilateral infiltrates.

B. *P. carinii* is most often seen in patients who are immunocompromised. *P. carinii* typically presents with a more indolent onset of several days to weeks time. The fevers are usually low-grade, and the sputum is usually not purulent. Chest X-ray is often normal, but can show patchy bilateral interstitial infiltrates.

C. *B. fragilis* is responsible for a significant number of anaerobic pulmonary infections. These infections are most often seen in patients who have aspirated, such as those with seizures or alcoholism. Aspiration pneumonia can involve any portion of the lung, but notoriously affects the right lower and middle lobes.

E. Pulmonary *B. anthracis* typically presents with a prodromal viral-like illness with myalgias, fatigue, and upper-respiratory infection-like symptoms that are then followed by rapid respiratory collapse. Chest X-ray classically shows widening of the mediastinum because of the associated lymphadenopathy.

97. **B.** There is much debate about the appropriate empiric antibiotic therapy for *Streptococcus pneumoniae*; however, of the choices listed, a third-generation cephalosporin would be best initially. Most practitioners would also start this patient on empiric macrolide therapy to treat for any possible "atypical" organism such as *Mycoplasma* or *Chlamydia*. However, this patient does not present with signs of infection by "atypical" organisms.

A. Clindamycin would be a good choice if you were treating an aspiration or anaerobic pneumonia, but that is not the case here.

C. Sulfamethoxazole-trimethoprim is the drug of choice for treatment of pneumonia caused by *P. carinii*; however, it is not appropriate for first-line therapy against pneumococcal disease in a sick patient.

D. Penicillin should not be used as first-line therapy against pneumococcal pneumonia because of the high resistance patterns that are present within some communities.

E. Amantadine can decrease the time course of some viral forms of pneumonia such as that caused by influenza A if it is initiated early in the course. However, it has no efficacy against pneumococcal disease.

98. **A.** Pleural effusions are divided into two major categories: exudative and transudative. *Transudative* effusions are the result of a pressure difference between the vasculature space and the surrounding tissue and pleural space. This pressure difference is from either a low oncotic pressure in the vasculature (such as a hypoalbuminemic state, which allows fluid to shift out of the vascular space and into the extravascular space), or high hydrostatic pressure (such as in congestive heart failure, which pushes the fluid out of the vascular space and into the extravascular space). In a transudative effusion, the vascular membrane remains intact, figuratively speaking. *Exudates* are the result of inflammation, usually from infection or malignancy, which weakens the vascular membrane and allows fluid and associated proteins to leak into the pleural space. Understanding this, one would expect to see *lower* levels of protein and LDH in the fluid if it were caused by pressure changes (i.e., transudative) and *higher* levels if it were caused by inflammatory changes (i.e., exudative). Light's criteria, which are based on these principles, are used to determine whether a pleural effusion is exudative or not. To be classified as an exudative effusion, *only one of the following three criteria must be met*:

- $TP_{effusion}/TP_{serum} > 0.5$
- $LDH_{effusion}/LDH_{serum} > 0.6$
- $LDH_{effusion} > 2/3$ the upper limit of normal LDH_{serum}

In this clinical case, one would expect that the patient has an inflammatory effusion as the result of his pneumonia (i.e., exudative). Of the choices listed, "A" is the only answer in which the above criteria are met.

B, C, D, E. See explanation for A.

99. **C.** This patient has the classic triad of Reiter's syndrome: conjunctivitis (or uveitis), urethritis, and arthritis. Reiter's syndrome is a type of reactive arthritis, which is a type of seronegative (rheumatoid factor-negative) spondylarthropathy. Other seronegative spondylarthropathies include ankylosing spondylitis, psoriatic arthritis, and inflammatory bowel disease-associated arthritis. To be diagnosed with "Reiter's," the patient must have all three portions of the triad. Patients with Reiter's syndrome are usually young men who present with an abrupt onset of monoarticular or asymmetric oligoarticular arthritis with a history of a preceding urethritis (often from *Chlamydia* infection) or diarrheal illness (often from *Shigella*, *Salmonella*, *Campylobacter*, or *Yersinia*). They have ocular disease ranging from a mild conjunctivitis to a severe uveitis. The arthritis usually involves the knee, ankle, or foot, but also may involve the wrist and fingers. This patient had a finding on his examination of dactylitis, or "sausage digit," which is seen in Figure 99. Dactylitis is seen most often in psoriatic arthritis and Reiter's syndrome. Our patient had no evidence of psoriasis. There are other clinical features that can help distinguish between the other types of arthritis given as possible answers.

A. Psoriatic arthritis is the other arthritis in the differential when a patient presents with a "sausage digit." It is important to look for evidence of subclinical skin disease, especially in places such as the scalp, umbilicus, and gluteal cleft. Most patients with psoriatic arthritis have obvious skin disease. Our patient did not have psoriasis and did have many of the findings of Reiter's syndrome.

B. Rheumatoid arthritis presents with symmetrical polyarthritis and is more common in women in this age group. Rheumatoid arthritis does not cause dactylitis as seen in our patient.

D. Gonococcal arthritis is more common in women than in men. It is abrupt in onset, and patients may have urethritis, although usually associated with a discharge in men. Gonococci are found on culture of the penile discharge. There is usually not a dactylitis, although tenosynovitis may be present. Patients also do not usually have conjunctivitis with gonococcal arthritis.

E. Osteoarthritis is a noninflammatory arthritis and is due to wear and tear of the cartilage of joints. It is mostly seen in the elderly and affects the distal phalangeal joints (with classic Heberden's and Bouchard's nodes) as well as the weight-bearing joints of the knees and hips. It is a gradual process and is not likely to be the cause of this patient's symptoms.

100. **D.** To date, only two clear predisposing factors have been identified for the development of a reactive arthritis or other seronegative (rheumatoid factor negative) spondylarthropathy: a preceding infection (enteric or GU) with a pathogen such as *Chlamydia*, *Shigella*, *Salmonella*, *Campylobacter*, or *Yersinia*, and the presence of HLA-B27. The presence of the HLA-B27 major histocompatibility complex (MHC) is the *most* important factor in determining the predisposition for developing a seronegative spondylarthropathy.

A. A culture of fluid aspirated from the joint may be positive in a patient who has septic arthritis, but it will be negative in patients who have reactive arthritis or Reiter's. The arthritis that develops in these latter conditions is the result of an autoimmune process, not an infectious one.

B. Rheumatoid factor can be positive in a host of autoimmune processes that can cause arthritis; however, one would not expect it to be positive in this case.

C. It is unusual for gonorrhea to cause urethritis without urethral discharge. In addition, reactive arthritis from gonococcal infection does not present with "sausage digits" as described in Table 99. Although he is at risk for contracting gonorrhea and should be tested, one would not expect this to be the cause of his symptoms.

E. Periosteal thickening and elevation along with bone erosion and soft tissue swelling are radiographic findings of osteomyelitis. Acute dactylitis usually presents radiographically with soft-tissue swelling alone.

101. A 24-year-old man presents with a history of increasing left knee pain and swelling for the past 3 days. He has had subjective fevers and is now unable to bear weight on his left knee. He denies any recent trauma and has never had an episode like this before. His past medical history is significant for hepatitis C, which he contracted by using IV drugs. On examination, he has a temperature of 101.6°F (38.7°C), a heart rate of 92, respiratory rate of 16, and blood pressure of 126/82. He is nontoxic in appearance, but is in a significant amount of pain. His examination is unremarkable with the exception of his left knee. There is marked swelling noted as depicted in Figure 101. He has no specific joint line tenderness or crepitus, but does have pain with passive flexion in the middle range of motion of his knee. You perform a diagnostic arthrocentesis at the bedside and obtain approximately 20 mL of yellow fluid that you send to the laboratory for immediate analysis. The following results are obtained: Color yellow and opaque; viscosity low; WBCs 108,800; PMNs 78%. Culture is pending, and crystal analysis is negative. Which of the following statements is most accurate?

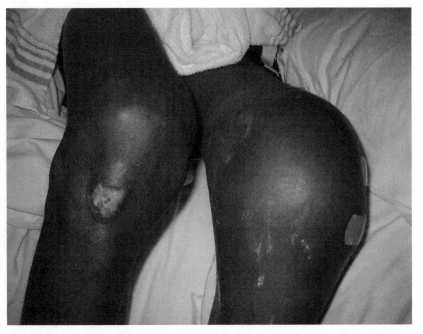

Figure 101 • Image courtesy of Dr. Brenda Shinar, Banner Good Samaritan Medical Center, Phoenix, Arizona

A. The patient likely has a septic arthritis and should be started on empiric IV antibiotic therapy while awaiting culture results
B. The patient likely has a septic arthritis and culture results should be obtained before starting IV antibiotics
C. The patient likely has an effusion secondary to trauma and should be observed until culture results are available
D. The patient likely has an inflammatory arthritis secondary to hepatitis C and should be started on intra-articular corticosteroid injections
E. The patient likely has a meniscal tear with an effusion. He should be given nonsteroidal anti-inflammatory drugs (NSAIDs) and an orthopedic referral

102. A 17-year-old woman presents with shortness of breath and a nonproductive cough that started approximately 12 hours before her arrival in the ED. In addition to shortness of breath, she complains of wheezing and chest tightness. She denies fever or chest pain. She was diagnosed with asthma when she was 10 years old and has had numerous exacerbations since that time. She has previously been admitted to the ICU for observation, but has never been intubated. Her home medication regimen includes inhaled albuterol, inhaled fluticasone, and oral montelukast. She also takes loratidine for seasonal allergy symptoms. On examination, you find her sitting in a tripod position on the bed speaking in short sentences. She is anxious with a respiratory rate of 26. Room-air oxygen saturation is 91%. She is afebrile with a heart rate of 88 and blood pressure of 116/74. Pulmonary examination reveals diffuse expiratory wheezes in all of her lung fields with diminished air exchange. The remainder of her examination is unremarkable. You obtain baseline labs, a chest x-ray, and a room-air arterial blood gas (ABG). Chest X-ray reveals mild flattening of the diaphragm bilaterally, but no focal infiltrates or abnormalities. She is started on continuous inhaled β-agonist therapy, oxygen supplementation, and IV corticosteroids. The results of the ABG drawn on room air show: pH 7.40; $paCO_2$ 42; paO_2 88; HCO_3^- = 22; oxygen saturation 92%. Which of the following statements is most accurate?

A. Her ABG is reassuring and she should be continued on her current medications and monitored
B. Her ABG shows an oxygenation problem and the focus of her care should be on improving her paO_2
C. Her ABG reveals a respiratory acidosis, which is expected in an acute exacerbation of asthma
D. Her ABG is worrisome and endotracheal intubation should be considered
E. Her ABG is normal and she can be discharged after she is given IV corticosteroids

---

The response options for items 103 through 108 are the same. You will be required to select one answer for each item in the set.

A. Transudative effusion in a patient with congestive heart failure (CHF)
B. Chylous effusion in a patient with lymphoma
C. Rheumatoid effusion in a patient with severe rheumatoid arthritis (RA)
D. Tuberculous effusion in a patient with primary tuberculosis (TB) and HIV
E. Empyema in a patient with *Streptococcus pneumoniae* pneumonia
F. Malignant effusion in a patient with metastatic squamous cell carcinoma
G. Pleural effusion secondary to pulmonary infarction resulting from a pulmonary embolism

For each of the pleural fluid findings, select the appropriate disease state (in each case the patient has a serum total protein of 7.0 g/dL and an LDH of 150 U/L).

103. Appearance thick, grayish-white; pH 6.9; LDH 2000 U/L; glucose 25 mg/dL; Gram stain reveals numerous neutrophils with gram-positive cocci in pairs

104. Appearance clear, yellow; pH 7.40; LDH 50 U/L; glucose 70 mg/dL; total protein 2.0 g/dL; Gram stain reveals no organisms

105. Appearance milky green; pH 7.0; LDH 1500 U/L; glucose 5 mg/dL; WBCs 500; 85% lymphocytes; triglycerides 30 mg/dL

106. Appearance straw-colored; pH 7.30; LDH 600 U/L; protein 5.5 g/dL; glucose 70 mg/dL; WBCs 4000; 60% lymphocytes

107. Appearance milky; pH 7.60; LDH 450; total protein 5.0 g/dL; WBCs 1000; 60% lymphocytes; triglycerides 120 mg/dL

108. Appearance bloody; pH 7.40; LDH 1000; total protein 4.5 g/dL; glucose 70 mg/dL; RBCs 10,000; WBCs 2000; eosinophils 15%

End of set

109. Light's criteria have been modified by Heffner et al. to allow clinicians to determine whether a patient has an exudative or a transudative pleural effusion without the need to get serum values simultaneously. Which of the following are the correct values used in the modified criteria?

A. Pleural fluid LDH >66% of serum upper limit of normal; pleural fluid cholesterol >45 mg/dL; or pleural fluid protein >2.9 g/dL

B. Pleural fluid LDH >45% of serum upper limit of normal; pleural fluid cholesterol >45 mg/dL; or pleural fluid protein >2.9 g/dL

C. Pleural fluid albumin >45% of serum upper limit of normal; pleural fluid cholesterol >100 mg/dL; or pleural fluid ANA >1:80 titer

D. Pleural fluid LDH >66% of serum upper limit of normal; pleural fluid triglyceride >110 mg/dL; or pleural fluid protein >5.0 g/dL

E. Pleural fluid LDH >45% of serum upper limit of normal; pleural fluid cholesterol >45 mg/dL; or pleural fluid albumin >4.0 g/dL

110. A 55-year-old man comes to your clinic with complaints of hemoptysis. He states that for the past month he has occasionally coughed up some sputum that is streaked with blood. This has never happened to him before. His past medical history is significant for 50 pack-years of tobacco abuse, high blood pressure, and diabetes type II. He denies fever, chest pain, and weight loss. Physical exam is normal. You order a chest X-ray and some baseline labs. His CBC reveals a normal WBC with a hemoglobin of 16 g/dL and a hematocrit of 48%. His chest X-ray reveals some hyperinflation and flattening of the diaphragms without any sign of infiltrate or mass. What is the most appropriate next step in the evaluation of his hemoptysis?

A. Order a sputum for cytology

B. Give the patient reassurance and advise him to stop smoking

C. Treat the patient empirically for acute bronchitis and have him follow up in 1 month

D. Order CT scan of the chest

E. Send the patient to a pulmonologist for a bronchoscopy

111. A 30-year-old woman comes to your office complaining of chronic coughing for the past month. She has never had problems with her lungs or smoked, but approximately 1 month ago she was working as a house cleaner and became acutely ill while cleaning a bathroom with a mixture of ammonia and bleach. The fumes made her very short of breath and wheezy and she was hospitalized for treatment and observation of her pulmonary status. Since that incident, she complains of recurrent cough and shortness of breath when she exercises and when she is exposed to cold air. On physical exam, her vital signs are normal. Her lung exam is clear with good air movement, and she does not wheeze on forced expiration. You send her for a chest X-ray and pulmonary function tests, which are normal. The patient insists that she has significant damage to her lungs, and that she has been harmed by this event. What is the next step in evaluation of her complaints?

A. Refer her to psychiatry for evaluation of post-traumatic stress disorder and anxiety
B. Reassure her that her pulmonary function tests and chest X-ray are normal and she does not need further testing
C. Obtain a room air arterial blood gas to look for an A-a gradient
D. Obtain pulmonary function tests with methacholine challenge to diagnose reversible reactive airway disease
E. Do pulse oximetry at rest and with exercise to determine whether she desaturates

---

The response options for items 112 through 116 are the same. You will be required to select one answer for each item in the set.

A. Right lower lobe consolidation due to streptococcal pneumonia
B. Right-sided pneumothorax
C. Left-sided pneumothorax
D. Right-sided pleural effusion
E. Left-sided pleural effusion
F. Severe obstructive lung disease due to emphysema
G. Impending respiratory failure
H. Acute asthma exacerbation

For each of the physical exam findings, select the appropriate diagnosis.

112. Right lower lobe bronchial breath sounds, egophony, and increased tactile fremitus

113. Right lower lobe decreased breath sounds, decreased tactile fremitus, and dullness to percussion

114. Bilateral decreased breath sounds, increased anteroposterior (AP) diameter of the chest, and prolonged expiration to inspiration ratio

115. Right lower lobe decreased breath sounds, hyperresonance to percussion, and trachea deviated to the left

116. Abdominal wall retraction during inspiration

End of set

The response options for items 117 through 120 are the same. You will be required to select one answer for each item in the set.

A. Spherocytes
B. Target cells
C. Tear drop cells
D. Schistocytes
E. Howell-Jolly bodies
F. Heinz bodies
G. Rouleaux formation

For each clinical scenario, select the appropriate finding on blood smear.

117. A 60-year-old man on quinine for leg cramps is brought to the ER for fever, headache, and visual changes and is found to be thrombocytopenic and anemic on his CBC.

118. A 60-year-old woman with a history of chronic lymphocytic leukemia has a hemoglobin of 8.0 g/dL and an LDH of 1000.

119. A 35-year-old woman with a history of sickle cell disease comes to the ER with a pain crisis.

120. A 45-year-old man with cirrhosis due to hepatitis C and a hemoglobin of 10 g/dL.

End of set

The next two questions (items 121 and 122) correspond to the following vignette.

A 38-year-old white man presents to your office with complaints of nasal congestion for 6 months. He states it started with a cold and the symptoms have not gotten better. He notes congestion with intermittent rhinorrhea. He denies any fevers, headache, or itchy and watery eyes. Past medical history is significant for hypertension, for which he takes a thiazide diuretic, and over-the-counter nasal medication that he takes three to four times a day as needed for his congestion. On exam he is afebrile and his vital signs are normal. In general, he is alert and in no acute distress. HEENT is significant for edematous nasal mucosa with clear rhinorrhea. The tympanic membranes are within normal limits and the oropharynx is without erythema or exudates. Chest is clear and heart exam is regular without murmur rub or gallop. Skin exam is normal.

121. What is the likely etiology of this man's congestion?

A. Allergic rhinitis
B. Foreign body
C. Nasal polyp
D. Vasomotor rhinitis
E. Rhinitis medicamentosa

122. What is the treatment for this patient's disorder?

    A. Inhaled nasal corticosteroids
    B. ENT evaluation
    C. Change hypertension medication to propanolol
    D. Discontinue inhaled nasal decongestant
    E. Nasal smear to check for eosinophils

End of set

---

123. A 35-year-old white man comes to your office with complaints of headache, congestion, and fever accompanied by purulent nasal drainage for 2 weeks. He states a history of recurrent sinus infections since he was young. He has a past medical history of allergic rhinitis, for which he takes an inhaled nasal corticosteroid. On review of systems he notes generalized fatigue. He denies any weight loss or gain. He tells you that he has frequent episodes of diarrhea that is watery and associated with bloating and flatulence. On exam, the patient's vital signs are within normal limits. In general he is alert, in no acute distress. His body mass index (BMI) is 17, and he is pale appearing. HEENT is significant for pink edematous nasal mucosa with purulent discharge. He has maxillary tenderness, right greater than left. His conjunctivae are pale. The rest of his exam is essentially normal except that his labs reveal iron-deficiency anemia. What immunodeficiency does this patient likely have?

    A. C5–C9 membrane attack complex (MAC) deficiency
    B. X-linked congenital agammaglobulinemia
    C. IgG deficiency
    D. IgA deficiency
    E. IgM deficiency

124. A 20-year-old Hispanic man presents to your office with swelling and induration on his left shoulder. He states that he received a tetanus booster yesterday. This hypersensitivity reaction is best described as:

    A. Immediate hypersensitivity
    B. Arthus type III reaction
    C. Delayed type IV reaction
    D. Late phase IgE-mediated reaction
    E. Anaphylaxis

> **The next two questions (items 125 and 126) correspond to the following vignette.**

A 23-year-old black woman with a history of asthma presents to your office as a new patient. She states she has never been hospitalized for her asthma but has made many ER visits (about 3 times per year). In an average week she uses her β-agonist inhaler three to four times. She awakens with nighttime cough every couple of weeks. Triggers include pets, colds, and allergies. She has never used any other medication.

125. This patient's asthma could be best described as:

A. Mild intermittent
B. Mild persistent
C. Moderate persistent
D. Severe
E. Exercise-induced

126. What is the best daily medical management for patients with this type of asthma?

A. Inhaled β-agonist only as needed
B. Inhaled β-agonist as needed and daily inhaled corticosteroid
C. No therapy needed
D. Long-acting β-agonist
E. Leukotriene receptor antagonist

End of set

---

127. A 24-year-old woman with a history of asthma since childhood presents to the ER with shortness of breath, which has been worsening over the past 3 days. On exam she is afebrile and tachypneic at 30 respirations per minute. Oxygen saturations are 99% on room air. She can converse with you in short phrases but appears to be in some respiratory distress. Her lung exam is significant for poor air movement and bilateral inspiratory and expiratory wheezes. There is also accessory muscle use noted. Your next step is to:

A. Draw an ABG, then intubate
B. Admit to the floor for observation
C. Inhaled corticosteroid therapy
D. One dose IV corticosteroid, then home on a steroid burst
E. Continuous inhaled β-agonist therapy and admit to ICU

> **The next two questions (items 128 and 129) correspond to the following vignette.**

A 45-year-old white man presents to your office with episodes of dry cough, malaise, and chills. He states this has been happening for the last few months. He recently moved with his family from the city to a farm to fulfill his lifelong dream of becoming a farmer. He denies any recent foreign travel or any known occupational or tuberculosis exposures. He denies hemoptysis, chest pain, or shortness of breath. He has noted some weight loss with a decrease in appetite. He recently visited his sister back in the city and noted that was the last time he felt well.

128. What is the likely antigen responsible for his symptoms?

A. Actinomycetes
B. Animal proteins
C. Fungi
D. Work-related chemicals
E. Arthropods

129. What is the optimal treatment for patients with hypersensitivity pneumonitis?

   A. Inhaled β-agonist therapy before known exposure
   B. High-dose IV steroids
   C. Antibiotic therapy
   D. Avoidance of antigen
   E. Short oral steroid bursts

End of set

130. An 18-year-old black woman presents to your office with recurrent episodes of leg and tongue swelling. She states these have been occurring for the last few years. She states that she will suddenly swell up without provocation. She denies any itching. She states her sister suffers from the same symptoms. Her immunodeficiency is best described as:

   A. C5–C9 MAC deficiency
   B. C3 deficiency
   C. C2 deficiency
   D. C1-esterase inhibitor deficiency
   E. IgA deficiency

131. A 36-year-old white woman in respiratory distress is brought to your ED by her friend, who states that they were at a picnic when the patient developed hives and difficulty breathing. They raced her to your ED. Your patient cannot communicate secondary to respiratory distress. Her friend thinks she has an allergy to bees. On physical exam she is afebrile, tachycardic at 130, blood pressure is 80/50, and saturations are 92% on room air. In general she is in moderate respiratory distress and she is diffusely erythematous with angioedema of her face and hands. Lungs are tight with wheezes throughout. Your next course in treatment is:

   A. IV epinephrine
   B. IV steroids
   C. Antihistamines
   D. Subcutaneous epinephrine
   E. Inhaled β-agonists

132. A 25-year-old white woman presents to your office for a new-patient visit. She denies any current complaints. On review of her past medical history she says that she had been hospitalized frequently as a child secondary to recurrent infections, in particular pneumonia. She was recently diagnosed with lupus. What laboratory test would be helpful in diagnosing her immunodeficiency?

   A. Serum immunoglobulins
   B. Nitroblue tetrazolium (NBT) dye reduction test
   C. Total hemolytic complement activity
   D. Anti-nuclear antibodies
   E. X chromosome inactivation analysis

> **The next two questions (items 133 and 134) correspond to the following vignette.**

A 71-year-old woman presents with complaints of bilateral hand pain that has been getting progressively worse over the past 6 months. She has also noticed increasing pain in her knees, with the right being worse than the left. She states she has approximately 10 minutes of morning stiffness each day and the pain seems worse after excessive activity. She denies any history of trauma or fevers. The joints in her hands and knees have not been red or swollen. The pain is most severe in her distal (DIP) and proximal (PIP) interphalangeal joints and her right knee. She has had no numbness or parasthesias. On examination, she is an obese woman in no acute distress. Her vital signs are normal, and she is afebrile. Her heart and lung examination is normal. Her abdomen is benign, and her neurologic examination is nonfocal. Her hands reveal full range of motion without evidence of effusions or erythema. There are nodules involving the DIP joints bilaterally. Her knee examination reveals full range of motion with bony enlargement over the medial aspect of both knees. In addition, there is significant crepitus noted with motion. She has no joint-line tenderness or effusions. You obtain X-rays of her hands and knees, which show osteophyte formation in both knees and in her DIP joints.

133. What is the most likely diagnosis?

   A. RA
   B. Systemic lupus erythematosus (SLE)
   C. Osteoarthritis (OA)
   D. Calcium pyrophosphate dihydrate (CPPD) deposition disease
   E. Reactive arthritis

134. Which of the following is the best initial treatment for this patient?

   A. Methotrexate
   B. Prednisone
   C. Allopurinol
   D. Ibuprofen
   E. Colchicine

End of set

> **The next three questions (items 135 through 137) correspond to the following vignette.**

A 48-year-old man presents to your clinic with complaints of severe right toe pain that began 36 hours ago. The pain is accompanied by redness and swelling in the toe. He does not recall any trauma to his toe, and there have been no prior occurrences. The patient reports subjective fevers, but has not objectively documented them. He states that the pain is so severe he cannot bear weight on his foot. He has no other medical problems. The only medication he takes is one aspirin a day. He does report ongoing IV drug use and drinks alcohol daily. On examination, he is afebrile with normal vital signs. His examination is essentially unremarkable with the exception of his right toe. There is marked swelling and redness over the first metatarsophalangeal joint and exquisite tenderness with minimal movement of the joint. His other joints appear normal on examination. You obtain labs and an X-ray of his right foot. The lab results show a normal WBC count and a uric acid level of 9.4 mg/dL. The X-rays of his right foot reveal soft-tissue swelling, but no bony changes. You then aspirate a small amount of fluid from the joint and send the specimen to the laboratory. The lab reports needle-like structures in the fluid that have strong negative birefringence.

135. What is the most likely cause of this patient's pain?

   A. Septic arthritis
   B. Gout
   C. CPPD
   D. Traumatic fracture
   E. SLE

136. Which of the following statements regarding the patient's uric acid level is true?

   A. It is normal, so gout can reliably be excluded
   B. It is normal, but gout cannot be excluded
   C. It is normal, making the diagnosis of CPPD more likely
   D. It is elevated, confirming the diagnosis of gout
   E. It is elevated, but cannot be used to make the diagnosis of gout

137. Which of the following would be the best choice for the initial treatment of this patient?

   A. Allopurinol
   B. Nafcillin
   C. Prednisone
   D. Indomethacin
   E. Immobilization with splints

End of set

> **The next three questions (items 138 through 140) correspond to the following vignette.**

A 40-year-old man presents with complaints of worsening low back pain over the past several weeks. The pain is mostly in his low back and gluteal areas. He states the pain is usually worse when he wakes up or after he has been resting for a while. As he becomes more active, the pain seems to diminish. He denies any trauma or heavy lifting. He has had no fevers, rashes, or pain in other joints. He says his diet is unchanged, and he has had no weight loss. Bowel habits are normal. He has no significant medical history and takes no regular medications. He is not sexually active but does use IV drugs occasionally. There has been no recent travel. On examination, his vital signs are normal and he is in no acute distress. His cardiovascular and lung exams are normal. His abdomen examination is benign, and his skin reveals no abnormal findings. Upon standing, he has noticeable stiffness and discomfort in his lower back area. He has no focal tenderness over his spinous processes. He has slightly limited range of motion in his lumbar spine. There is tenderness over his sacroiliac region. His straight-leg raise test is negative. His muscle strength, deep-tendon reflex, and sensory testing are all normal. You obtain blood work and X-rays of his lumbosacral spine. The X-rays show squaring and increased density anteriorly of the vertebral bodies. The sacroiliac joint margins are blurred with evidence of erosions.

138. What is the most likely diagnosis?

   A. Vertebral osteomyelitis
   B. Ankylosing spondylitis (AS)
   C. Reactive arthritis
   D. RA
   E. Inflammatory bowel disease (IBD)

139. Testing for which of the following will most likely yield a positive result in this patient?

   A. HLA-B27
   B. Blood culture
   C. Rheumatoid factor
   D. Anti-nuclear antibody
   E. Stool guaiac

140. In addition to spinal cord injuries, patients with this disease are at increased risk for the development of which complication?

   A. Nephritis
   B. Serositis
   C. Cerebritis
   D. Cutaneous lesions
   E. Uveitis

End of set

> **The next two questions (items 141 and 142) correspond to the following vignette.**

A 74-year-old woman presents to the ED complaining of a headache and fatigue that started approximately 24 hours ago. She has no prior history of migraines and states the pain is worse over the right side of her head. She denies focal weakness or slurred speech, but does report that her jaw becomes painful when eating. She also has noticed visual changes that she describes as "a black curtain starting to cover my vision." She also reports progressive pain in her shoulders and hips with morning stiffness, but denies chest pain or claudication of the arm. On examination, you find a pleasant, elderly woman in no acute distress. She has marked visual field defects in her right eye, but her left eye is normal. Funduscopic examination of the left eye is normal and the right eye reveals a swollen, pale disc with blurred margins. The remainder of her neurologic examination is normal with the exception of pain in her shoulders and hips bilaterally. Her cardiovascular examination is normal, and she has strong peripheral pulses bilaterally. Lungs are clear to auscultation, and abdomen is benign. Laboratory studies reveal normal CBC, renal function, and electrolytes.

141. Which of the following is the most likely cause of her symptoms?

A. Takayasu's arteritis
B. Cerebrovascular accident (CVA)
C. Temporal arteritis
D. SLE
E. Acute aortitis

142. Which of the following is the most appropriate next step in the management of this patient?

A. Obtain arteriography and initiate steroid therapy
B. Obtain anti-nuclear antibodies and initiate prednisone therapy
C. Obtain a CT scan of the brain and initiate antiplatelet therapy
D. Obtain a biopsy of temporal artery and initiate prednisone
E. Obtain rapid plasma reagin (RPR) results and initiate intramuscular penicillin therapy

End of set

> **The next three questions (items 143 through 145) correspond to the following vignette.**

A 45-year-old woman with RA presents to your clinic for routine follow-up. She was diagnosed approximately 9 years ago and has had a rapidly progressive disease course. She has morning stiffness for approximately one hour every morning, and she has suboptimal pain control. Most of her pain involves bilateral proximal interphalangeal (PIP) and metacarpophalangeal (MCP) joints. She is known to have high titers of rheumatoid factor (RF). Her treatment regimen consists of oral prednisone 20 mg daily and methotrexate 7.5 mg weekly. Entanercept was recently initiated at a dose of 25 mg subcutaneously twice weekly. On examination, she is afebrile and has normal vital signs. Head and neck exam are normal. Heart and lung examination are unremarkable. Her spleen is enlarged, nontender, and easily palpated when examining her abdomen. Her skin exam reveals rheumatoid nodules on the extensor surface of her forearms. Joint exam reveals moderate synovitis in the PIP and MCP joints diffusely. You are concerned that she has developed Felty's syndrome, so you order appropriate laboratory studies.

143. Which of the following abnormalities would support the diagnosis of Felty's syndrome?

A. Uremia
B. Prolonged partial thromboplastin time (aPTT)
C. Elevated aspartate aminotransferase (AST)
D. Neutropenia
E. Direct hyperbilirubinemia

144. Which of the following is a common extra-articular manifestation of RA?

A. Peptic ulcer disease
B. Pericardial effusion
C. Autoimmune hemolytic anemia
D. Nephrotic syndrome
E. Spontaneous pneumothorax

145. Methotrexate has many side effects. Patients are given folate to help prevent some of these side effects. Which of the following side effects of methotrexate may be ameliorated by the addition of folate to the patient's medication regimen?

A. Rash
B. Stomatitis
C. Pneumonitis
D. Liver transaminitis
E. Teratogenicity

End of set

146. A 32-year-old Hispanic woman presents with 5 weeks of fatigue, generalized weakness, and pallor. She denies fever, chills, or weight loss, but has had two urinary tract infections in the last month. She works in a factory that makes tires, but is unsure what chemicals are used at her workplace. Physical examination reveals pale conjunctivae and mucous membranes, heart rate of 95, but otherwise normal cardiovascular and pulmonary examinations. There is no palpable lymphadenopathy. Abdominal examination is benign with no evidence of hepatosplenomegaly. A CBC is obtained with the following results: WBC 2000/μL; differential: 60% neutrophils, 30% lymphocytes, 6% monocytes, remainder eosinophils and basophils. Hemoglobin level is 9.2 g/dL; hematocrit 29%; mean corpuscular volume (MCV) 85 fL; platelet count 45,000/μL, reticulocytes 0.5%. A bone marrow aspirate is obtained showing all cell lines to be hypocellular with an increase in fat cells. The diagnosis most consistent with this patient's presentation is:

A. Myelodysplastic syndrome
B. Aplastic anemia
C. Paroxysmal nocturnal hemoglobinuria
D. Chronic myelogenous leukemia
E. Folate deficiency

147. A 60-year-old woman presents with a new deep venous thrombosis (DVT). She denies any trauma, recent travel, or family history of hypercoagulable states. She is not a smoker and has no other significant medical history. Additional history is notable only for pruritus in the morning, noted after her showers. Vital signs include pulse 82, respiratory rate 18, oxygen saturation 98% on room air, and blood pressure 121/83. Physical examination is remarkable for facial plethora, spleen tip palpable 4 cm below the left costal margin, and normal cardiovascular and pulmonary examinations. Labs show the following results: Hemoglobin is 18 g/dL; hematocrit 52%. Which of the following statements is true concerning polycythemia vera?

A. A serum erythropoietin level of greater than 30 U/L is diagnostic of polycythemia vera
B. RBC mass studies are not useful in confirming the diagnosis of polycythemia vera
C. Phlebotomy is the treatment of choice and should be done until the patient develops an iron-deficiency anemia
D. Splenomegaly is not a common physical exam finding in polycythemia vera and should alert the physician to investigate for an underlying leukemia
E. WBC and platelet counts are typically normal in polycythemia vera

148. A 24-year-old man with Crohn's disease presents with 1 month of progressive fatigue and weakness. He currently takes sulfasalazine and recently completed a course of oral steroids. Vital signs include a pulse of 90, respiratory rate of 16, blood pressure of 110/75, and oxygen saturation of 98% on room air. Physical examination reveals pale mucous membranes, tachycardia with an otherwise normal cardiovascular examination, diffuse tenderness to palpation on abdominal examination, without palpable hepatosplenomegaly. A CBC with peripheral smear is obtained. The peripheral smear is shown in Figure 148. This patient's anemia is most likely due to:

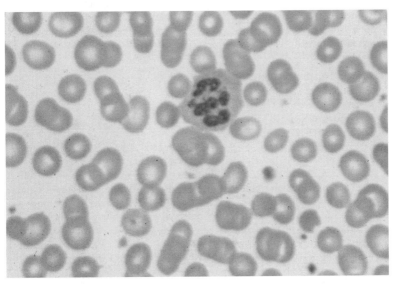

Figure 148 • Image courtesy of Dr. Brenda Shinar, Banner Good Samaritan Medical Center, Phoenix, Arizona

    A. Iron deficiency
    B. Blood loss
    C. Chronic disease
    D. B_{12} deficiency
    E. Folate deficiency

149. You are in clinic and seeing a patient with the diagnosis of "anemia" who has been placed on iron therapy empirically. You are unsure if the patient truly has iron deficiency or whether the problem is really anemia of chronic disease when you look through the chart. Which of the following statements is true regarding iron-deficiency anemia?

    A. Iron studies will show a low iron, low total iron-binding capacity, and high ferritin
    B. The most common cause of iron-deficiency anemia is decreased iron intake
    C. An increase in hemoglobin by 2 g/dL over 4 weeks of treatment is considered an acceptable response to iron therapy
    D. Pica is an uncommon symptom of untreated iron-deficiency anemia
    E. Ferritin levels are not affected by acute illness

150. A 17-year-old previously healthy woman presents to your office after being told she has anemia at a sports preparticipation screening. She reports occasional right upper quadrant pain after large meals, but is otherwise asymptomatic. Family history is remarkable for a mother with anemia. Physical examination is notable for splenomegaly, but otherwise is normal. Laboratory studies include: Hemoglobin 9.2 g/dL; MCV 85 fL; reticulocytes 7%; total bilirubin 3.4 mg/dL. The peripheral smear is shown in Figure 150. The next most appropriate step in management would be:

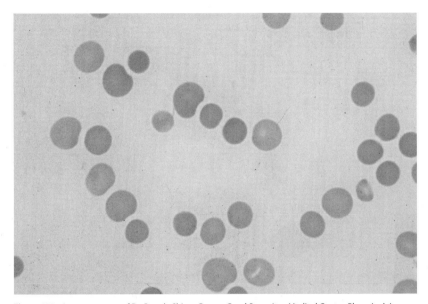

Figure 150 • Image courtesy of Dr. Brenda Shinar, Banner Good Samaritan Medical Center, Phoenix, Arizona

A. Bone marrow biopsy
B. Osmotic fragility test
C. Quantitative G6PD levels
D. Splenectomy
E. Obtain IgG and IgM autoantibody levels

Answers and Explanations

THREE

Answer Key

101.	A	118.	A	135.	B
102.	D	119.	E	136.	E
103.	E	120.	B	137.	D
104.	A	121.	E	138.	B
105.	C	122.	D	139.	A
106.	D	123.	D	140.	E
107.	B	124.	B	141.	C
108.	G	125.	B	142.	D
109.	B	126.	B	143.	D
110.	E	127.	E	144.	B
111.	D	128.	A	145.	B
112.	A	129.	D	146.	B
113.	D	130.	D	147.	C
114.	F	131.	A	148.	D
115.	B	132.	C	149.	C
116.	G	133.	C	150.	B
117.	D	134.	D		

101. **A.** This patient has clinical findings concerning for septic arthritis: fever, arthralgia, and pain with passive motion of the joint. In addition, the results of his arthrocentesis suggest an infectious process (Table 101). Once a bacterial infection has developed in a joint space, treatment must be initiated rapidly to prevent destruction of the joint. Given that he likely has a septic arthritis, he should be started on empiric IV antibiotic therapy as soon as possible and before culture results are available.

■ TABLE 101	Arthrocentesis Results			
	Normal	**Inflammatory**	**Septic**	**Hemorrhagic**
Volume (mL)	<3.5	>3.5	>3.5	>3.5
Color	Clear	Yellow	Yellow/green	Red
Clarity	Clear	Clear to opaque	Opaque	Bloody
Viscosity	High	Low	Low to high	Low to high
WBCs	<200	2000–10,000	>100,000	200–2000
PMNs	<25%	>50%	>75%	50–75%

B. As in the explanation for A, antibiotic therapy should not be withheld in a case of suspected septic arthritis because of the increased risk of joint destruction. You should start empiric therapy and modify this once culture results are available.

C. Traumatic effusions are usually not inflammatory (immune mediated). Occasionally, they are hemorrhagic, which will be evident by gross visualization of the fluid.

D. Although hepatitis C can cause arthralgias, it is not common to see large effusions associated with it. In addition, the synovial fluid would have a more inflammatory than septic appearance (Table 101).

E. The patient gives no history of trauma, and the fluid that was aspirated is significantly inflamed, which suggests infection. Patients with meniscal tears typically can state the time and place of their injury and should not have fever or the other indicators of an infected joint.

102. | **D.** This patient is in the midst of a serious asthma exacerbation. She is anxious, dyspneic, and tachypneic. She is sitting in a tripod position trying to breath easier, and she is becoming hypoxemic. All are warning signs for impending respiratory failure. In the initial phase of an acute exacerbation of asthma, the minute ventilation (respiratory rate × tidal volume) increases. As the minute ventilation increases, more CO_2 is exhaled and the $paCO_2$ should decrease. Therefore, you should not expect to see a normal $paCO_2$ in a patient who is compensating well for their acute attack. As our patient's exacerbation persisted, she has became more fatigued and, as a result, the tidal volumes she was able to generate became progressively smaller. As the tidal volumes decreased, she was unable to increase her respiratory rate any further and her minute ventilation began to decrease and $paCO_2$ to rise. Therefore, the "normal" $paCO_2$ obtained during her acute attack of asthma is worrisome because it is suggests that the $paCO_2$ is on an upward trend. This patient is becoming fatigued and is on the verge of respiratory failure. She should be considered for endotracheal intubation before a complete respiratory collapse occurs.

A, E. Her ABG appears normal, but it is not reassuring. Recognizing this subtlety can help you intervene more rapidly before the patient becomes unstable.

B. Although her oxygenation status is suboptimal, it is not the primary problem. It is a result of her ventilation problem. Although supplemental oxygen should be provided, further correction of her paO_2 is not our primary concern.

C. Although she is likely to develop respiratory acidosis if her condition continues to deteriorate, she has not yet become acidemic, as indicated by her neutral pH.

103. | **E.** Light's criteria help to diagnose pleural fluid as transudative or exudative. If any one of the three criteria is positive, then the fluid is an exudate. These criteria are: 1) A pleural fluid protein to serum protein ratio of >0.5, 2) a pleural fluid LDH to serum LDH ratio of >0.6, or 3) a pleural fluid LDH >2/3 the upper limit of normal serum LDH. This effusion is thick, grayish-white in color, which is probably pus. The pH is acidic, and the glucose is low along with a high LDH. Most importantly, the Gram stain is positive for organisms, which makes this an empyema. This effusion will need to be drained with a chest tube, and the patient may need to go to decortication to treat the infection.

104. | **A.** This effusion is a transudate, because the pH is normal, the pleural fluid protein to serum protein ratio is 0.28, and the pleural fluid LDH to serum LDH ratio is 0.33.

105. **C.** This effusion is due to RA. First, by analysis of the protein and LDH ratios, it is an exudate. It is milky green, which might confuse you into thinking that this is a chylous effusion; however, the triglycerides are <50 mg/dL, which virtually excludes a chylous effusion. Also, the glucose is extremely low, at 5 mg/dL, which is most commonly seen with rheumatoid effusions. The WBC count is not very high, but is mostly lymphocytic, which also goes along with a rheumatoid-related effusion.

106. **D.** This effusion is consistent with a tuberculous effusion (which needs to be distinguished from a tuberculous empyema). Tuberculous effusions are caused by a delayed hypersensitivity reaction to the AFB antigen, which may leak into the pleural space. They are usually straw-colored and exudative. The pH may be low (around 7.30) and the glucose may be low, but not as low as in a tuberculous empyema or a rheumatic effusion. The white cells are predominantly lymphocytic, and there is usually a paucity (<5%) of mesothelial cells in TB effusions.

107. **B.** Chylous effusions are turbid or milky-appearing because of their high lipid content and are usually a result of a thoracic duct disruption. Causes of this disruption can be traumatic or nontraumatic. The most common nontraumatic cause is a lymphoma in the chest. Other nontraumatic causes include sarcoidosis or tuberculosis. Traumatic causes are most often related to surgeries of the chest. A triglyceride content in the effusion of >110 mg/dL strongly suggests a chylous effusion, whereas a triglyceride content of <30 mg/dL virtually rules out the diagnosis. It the content falls between these two numbers, then a lipoprotein analysis should be done on the fluid. If chylomicrons are found, then the diagnosis of a chylous effusion can be made.

108. **G.** An eosinophilic pleural effusion can have many causes. It may be associated with a pneumothorax, a hemothorax, a pulmonary infarction, a parasitic or tuberculous infection; it can also be drug-induced. This pleural effusion was bloody, and it was exudative, making the best choice of answers "G."

   F. An effusion related to metastatic cancer lung cancer will most likely be exudative and is often grossly bloody. The cytology may be helpful if it is positive, but if negative, the sensitivity of cytology is not good enough to rule out cancer.

109. **B.** The values as given by Heffner et al. (*Chest*, 1997;111:970–980) are convenient to use because they eliminate the need for drawing a patient's serum at the same time (or as close as possible to the same time) as performing a thoracentesis. Remember, just as in Light's criteria, if just *one* of the criteria is met, the pleural effusion is considered an exudate. The criteria are: Pleural fluid LDH >45% of the serum upper limit of normal; pleural fluid cholesterol >45 mg/dL; or pleural fluid total protein >2.9 gm/dL. There is no albumin, ANA, or triglyceride in the Heffner criteria of transudate vs. exudative pleural effusion.

   A, C, D, E. These values are incorrect. See explanation for B.

110. E. Studies have shown that small endobronchial cancerous lesions may be found as a cause for hemoptysis in patients with clear chest X-rays between 0% and 20% of the time. Factors that increase the risk for occult malignancy in patients with hemoptysis and a clear chest X-ray include cigarette smoking, age >40 years, and hemoptysis that continues for longer than 1 week. Because lung cancer may be resectable in its early stages, it is important to look for it. In this patient, who is 55 years old with a significant smoking history and the hemoptysis lasting a month, the most appropriate next step is to refer him to a pulmonologist for a bronchoscopy.

A. Sputum for cytology would be helpful if it were positive, because the next step would be to go to bronchoscopy to look for the source of malignant cells. However, sputum cytology is not sufficiently sensitive, and many small cancers can be missed. Therefore, it is not the appropriate next step for this patient.

B. It is always important to advise patients who smoke of the risks to their health, and to encourage them to quit; however, it is not appropriate to give this patient reassurance regarding his hemoptysis.

C. In a patient who is at low risk for occult malignancy, such as a younger patient, one who does not smoke, or one who presents with upper respiratory symptoms and a cough with minimal streaks of hemoptysis, it may be appropriate to treat for empiric bronchitis to see if the hemoptysis resolves. However, that is not the correct choice for management in this patient scenario.

D. A *high-resolution* CT scan of the chest may be an alternative to a fiberoptic bronchoscopy in a patient for whom bronchoscopy is contraindicated (such as patients with bleeding disorders). However, a plain CT scan is not appropriate. A high-resolution CT scan takes coronal slices through the chest at smaller intervals than a normal CT scan and is more sensitive for smaller lesions. Bronchoscopy, however, is preferred for both diagnosis and cost-effectiveness

111. D. Asthma is a combination of bronchial hyperreactivity, constriction, and chronic inflammation. There are many causes of occupational asthma, including metal salts, wood and vegetable dusts, industrial chemicals and plastics, and others. There are probably three separate mechanisms for this type of asthma: 1) the agent may trigger an IgE antibody resulting in immunologic sensitization; 2) the substance itself can release factors that cause bronchoconstriction; and 3) the substance can cause a direct or a reflex stimulation of the airways in latent (or already diagnosed) asthmatics. The methacholine challenge is the appropriate test to evaluate this patient, to see whether she develops signs of airway bronchoconstriction and obstruction on pulmonary function tests when exposed to methacholine. A negative challenge (the FEV_1 remains 80% or greater than predicted) in a patient not on anti-asthma medications excludes the diagnosis of asthma with 95% certainty.

A. This patient should not be referred to psychiatry, because you have not eliminated reactive airway disease as a diagnosis based on the tests that you have performed.

B. Patients with asthma may have completely normal chest X-rays and pulmonary function tests when they are not in an acute attack. This patient needs a methacholine challenge before asthma can be ruled out.

C. A room-air arterial blood gas would not help make the diagnosis of asthma in this patient who is currently asymptomatic.

E. Oxygen desaturation with exercise is a sensitive indicator of gas exchange abnormalities, but is not specific. It will not help make the diagnosis of asthma in this patient. Oxygen desaturation with exercise may be pronounced in patients with HIV and *Pneumocystis carinii* pneumonia (PCP), patients with early interstitial lung disease, and pulmonary vascular disease, such as primary pulmonary hypertension.

112. A. This patient has bronchial breath sounds in the right lower lobe. (Bronchial breath sounds are synonymous with "tubular" and "tracheal" breath sounds.) These sounds are different from the usual alveolar sounds that are heard in the periphery of the lung. If you listen to a normal chest at either lower lobe, you will hear a fine noise on inspiration and nothing on expiration. If you listen over the trachea, you will hear a loud noise during inspiration *and* expiration. The noise that you hear over the trachea is *abnormal* to hear in the lung periphery, and it means that large airway noises are being transmitted to the periphery. This is usually because the alveoli are full of a material (fluid, pus) and are consolidating the lobe. (Bronchial breath sounds can also be heard when large effusions "squish" the lung parenchyma and allow the large airway noise to be heard in the periphery, but usually effusions cause decreased breath sounds.) Egophony is also heard with consolidation. With your stethoscope over the area of consolidation, ask the patient to say "eeeeee"; the sound will change to "aayyyy." Increased tactile fremitus is seen in consolidation as well. To test for this, you should place your hands *firmly* against the patient's back or chest wall (or you can alternate the same hand back and forth, like your stethoscope) and have the patient say "ninety-nine" over and over again. You will sense an increased vibration over the area of consolidated lung, meaning that there is a direct, solid communication from the bronchus, through the lung, and out to the chest wall—a sign of consolidation.

113. D. This patient has decreased breath sounds over the right lower lobe. The next step in evaluating the pathology is palpation to determine whether it is dull or hyperresonant. The dullness signifies either an effusion or consolidation of the lobe. The decreased tactile fremitus indicates a probable effusion between the lung tissue and the chest wall, as opposed to a consolidation, which would cause *increased* tactile fremitus.

114. F. This patient has decreased breath sounds bilaterally. The increased AP diameter of the chest (also known as a "barrel chest") implies chronic air trapping. The long expiration to inspiration ratio suggests obstruction to air flow, which is seen in patients with chronic obstructive lung disease or asthma. However, the barrel shape of the chest makes you think that this is something more chronic and long-standing than an asthma exacerbation, and severe obstructive lung disease due to emphysema is the correct answer.

115. **B.** This patient has decreased breath sounds over the right lung; however, he is hyperresonant to percussion, which should make you think of a pneumothorax. The trachea is deviated *away* from the pneumothorax, because the large volume of air in the pleural space is pushing it away. A large right-sided pleural effusion also may deviate the trachea to the left (as would anything with high volume), but there would be dullness, and not hyperresonance, to percussion.

116. **G.** The abdominal wall usually expands with inspiration. This patient's abdomen is retracting with inspiration, which is called respiratory paradox. The most common reason for this is a patient who is becoming severely tired from respiratory effort, and the diaphragm is being pulled upward as the intercostal muscles do all the work of breathing. Respiratory alternans is seen when a patient has normal abdominal wall expansion with breathing that alternates with paradoxical abdominal wall movement. Both of these scenarios are serious and indicate impending respiratory failure.

C. The left-sided pneumothorax would have the same findings as "B," but on the left side.

E. The left-sided effusion would have the same findings as in "D," but on the left side.

117. **D.** This patient is presenting with four of the five classic signs of thrombotic thrombocytopenic purpura (TTP): fever, neurologic changes, anemia, and thrombocytopenia. In addition, he takes a medication, quinine, known to have a rare side effect of TTP. TTP is a disorder of endothelial injury that causes the activation of platelets (and thrombocytopenia) and the formation of fibrin strands within blood vessels. The fibrin strands shear the RBCs, resulting in a microangiopathic hemolytic anemia. Schistocytes are fragmented RBCs seen on the blood smears of patients with microangiopathic hemolytic anemias such as TTP, hemolytic uremic syndrome (HUS), and the hemolysis, elevated liver enzymes, low platelet (HELLP) syndrome of pregnancy.

118. **A.** Spherocytes are seen in the peripheral smears of patients with autoimmune hemolytic anemias (AIHAs). In this anemia, the patient forms antibodies to the RBC membrane; in the spleen, a "bite" of the membrane is taken out, effectively giving the cell a "facelift" and changing its shape from a biconcave disk to a sphere. Patients with chronic lymphocytic leukemia are prone to the development of AIHA.

119. **E.** Howell-Jolly bodies are nuclear remnants that are left in the circulating RBCs of patients who have had their spleen removed or have functional asplenia. The spleens of patients with sickle cell disease have usually infarcted by late childhood; these patients will be functionally asplenic.

120. **B.** Target cells are formed when the RBC has an increased surface area (membrane) to volume (cytoplasm) ratio. Any process that increases the amount of cell membrane or decreases the amount of cytoplasm will cause a target cell. Chronic liver disease causes target cells by increasing the amount of phospholipids deposited in the cell membrane (thereby increasing the ratio), and thalassemia and severe iron deficiency cause target cells by decreasing the cytoplasmic volume (which also increases the ratio).

C. Tear drop cells are seen in myelofibrosis.

F. Heinz bodies are aggregates of denatured hemoglobin and are most often seen in glucose 6-phosphate dehydrogenase (G6PD) deficiency and in thalassemias.

G. Rouleaux formation is seen on the peripheral smear in approximately 50% of patients with multiple myeloma. It consists of RBCs that appear in stacks, like coins.

121. **E.** Rhinitis medicamentosa can occur with many drugs, but the most common precipitant is over-the-counter sympathomimetic nasal sprays used to treat congestion. When used for several days, one can develop rebound congestion when the medication wears off. The patient often starts to use more of the nasal spray at higher doses, which then begins a vicious cycle.

A. Allergic rhinitis is usually seasonal and accompanied by other symptoms such as watery, itchy eyes and sneezing. Patients give a history of worsening symptoms at different times of the year. Common allergens include dust mites and animal proteins. People typically give a personal or family history of rhinitis, eczema, or asthma. Exam is significant for turbinate edema with pallor or a bluish hue. This patient does not give any temporal relationship to symptoms, and his exam is more consistent with nonallergic rhinitis.

B. This patient does not give any history of placing or inserting foreign objects in his nose, a very common occurrence in children. Physical exam is often significant for unilateral congestion (where foreign object is located) and purulent discharge.

C. Nasal polyps are associated with chronic allergic rhinitis. On exam they are pale, polypoid masses that are insensitive to pain. Treatment begins with nasal steroids, but if the patient is still symptomatic, surgery can be performed.

D. Vasomotor rhinitis is chronic nasal congestion worsened by changes in temperature and humidity and with new odors. Physical exam is significant for pink, boggy nasal mucosa. Nasal itching is very rare, as is the presence of eosinophils, which are common in allergic rhinitis. Avoidance of triggers and inhaled nasal steroids aid in treatment.

122. **D.** This man has rhinitis medicamentosa caused by continual use of a sympathomimetic nasal spray. His symptoms worsen when the medication wears off and thus begins the vicious cycle. Treatment is removal of the offending agent. Nasal corticosteroids have been used with some improvement. Symptoms can remain for up to 1 year.

A. Inhaled nasal corticosteroids are used primarily in the treatment of allergic rhinitis. They can also be used with rhinitis medicamentosa, but studies have shown only some improvement in symptoms.

B. ENT evaluation at this point is unnecessary, given the patient history and physical exam. It is unlikely that he is suffering from nasal tumor or foreign body.

C. Antihypertensives are known to cause rhinitis. The main offending agent is propanolol. Thiazides are less likely to cause rhinitis.

E. A nasal smear to check for eosinophils would help differentiate allergic rhinitis from nonallergic rhinitis. Because this patient does not have allergy-type symptoms, this is not necessary.

123. **D.** IgA deficiency is the most common immunoglobulin deficiency with an incidence reaching 1/600 in white populations. This patient gives a history of recurrent sinopulmonary infections and intermittent diarrhea, which are consistent with IgA deficiency. There is a concordance with IgA deficiency and celiac sprue, and this patient has diarrhea and iron-deficiency anemia, which should make you think of celiac disease. Another manifestation of IgA deficiency includes anaphylactic reactions to blood transfusions. The diagnosis is made by measuring quantitative IgA levels. Treatment includes prophylactic antibiotics to lessen the number of infections. If this does not help, IV immune globulin (IVIG) has been tried with some success.

A. C5–C9 MAC deficiency is also called terminal complement deficiency. Complement proteins C5 through C9 are responsible for the membrane attacking complex after initiation of the immune response by antibodies in both the classic and alternative activation cascades. Deficiency of these proteins leads to increased infections with *Neisseria* species including both meningococcal and gonococcal infections. This patient does not give this type of history.

B. X-linked agammglobulinemia presents in males, usually ages 6 to 18 months, with recurrent sinopulmonary infections secondary to *Staphylococcus*, *Streptococcus*, and meningococcus. There are no B cells present in serum. These patients have normal resistance to viral illnesses, fungi, and gram-negative organisms. If caught early, prognosis is good with IVIG treatment.

C. IgG deficiency is also known as common variable hypogammaglobulinemia. Patients have decreased resistance to encapsulated organisms such as *Streptococcus pneumoniae* and *Haemophilus influenzae*. Peak incidence occurs between 25 and 40 years of age. Clinical manifestations include recurrent sinopulmonary infections, recurrent enteroviral infections, and an association with autoimmune disorders and rheumatologic disorders. Treatment is IVIG over 2 to 4 weeks.

E. IgM deficiency is also known as Wiskott-Aldrich syndrome. Patients often present in infancy with thrombocytopenia, recurrent sinopulmonary infections, eczema, and other autoimmune disorders. IgM levels are generally low. Treatment includes bone marrow transplant, IVIG, splenectomy, and prophylactic antibiotics.

124. **B.** Arthus (hypersensitivity type III) reactions are mediated by IgG antibodies, which form complexes with antigens. These hypersensitivity reactions are less common than IgE-mediated hypersensitivity reactions. Arthus reactions are described as deposition of immune complexes that cause a localized inflammatory reaction. They occur about 8 to 24 hours after inoculation. An antigen that has been injected (in this case the tetanus vaccine) stimulates this patient's localized immune response. This will not progress on to anaphylaxis.

A. Immediate hypersensitivity occurs within 1 hour of exposure to an allergen. Typically allergens include stings, drugs, and foods. Urticaria and hives are initial presenting signs that can advance to anaphylaxis. This reaction is IgE mediated.

C. Delayed type IV reactions are mediated by T cells, not antibodies. They typically occur 24 to 48 hours after exposure. Exposure to mycobacterial proteins or poison ivy are examples of type IV reactions. Reactions are typically local, with erythema, induration, and dermatitis present.

D. Late-phase IgE-mediated reactions present as local erythema, burning, and induration typically seen with reactions to local skin testing. The reaction is secondary to mast cell release.

E. Anaphylaxis is an extreme form of immediate hypersensitivity reaction that is usually IgE mediated. There are non-IgE mediated forms of anaphylaxis secondary to release of cytoplasmic granules. These are called "anaphylactoid" reactions. An example of an anaphylactoid reaction is the usual reaction to radiocontrast dye.

125. **B.** This patient's asthma can best be described as mild persistent. Mild persistent asthma is defined as having symptoms more than once per week that require bronchodilators, nighttime awakening once every 2 weeks, and fluctuations in peak flows of 20% or more.

A. Mild intermittent asthma criteria include symptoms two times or fewer in a week, fewer than two nighttime awakenings per month, and peak flows consistently above 80%.

C. Moderate persistent asthma is defined as daily symptoms with bronchodilator use, at least one nighttime awakening per week, and peak flows ranging from 60% to 80% of predicted values.

D. Severe asthma is defined as symptoms with any trigger, usually occurring daily and requiring use of a bronchodilator. Awakening four to seven times nightly and peak flows less than 60% of predicted normal values are also criteria for severe asthma.

E. Exercise-induced asthma usually falls into the mild intermittent category, because symptoms are usually only related to exercise and peak flows remain greater than 80% of predicted values.

126. **B.** The initiation of an anti-inflammatory agent is indicated in cases of mild-persistent asthma. In this case, the patient would most likely benefit from an inhaled corticosteroid. She should use an inhaled β-agonist as needed for rescue purposes. This therapy should lower the number of symptomatic episodes she has per week.

A. An inhaled β-agonist would not be adequate therapy for this patient. This would treat only the acute symptoms, which she is having quite frequently. There would be no therapy for the underlying inflammation in her bronchioles.

C. This patient requires medical therapy on an outpatient basis. Not treating her would be a medical liability.

D. A long-acting β-agonist is often added to therapy of patients with moderate persistent and severe asthma. It cuts down on the number of short-acting β-agonists needed. It does not treat the inflammatory component of asthma.

E. Leukotriene receptor antagonists inhibit leukotrienes, which are released during asthma exacerbations. Leukotrienes are responsible for airway edema, mucus secretion, and bronchoconstriction that especially awaken the patient at night, because they are the late-phase mediators of inflammation. These antagonists can be started in patients with mild persistent asthma after initiation of β-agonist and corticosteroid therapy, but are more frequently used in patients with moderate to severe asthma.

127. **E.** This patient is very ill, as witnessed on her physical exam (in particular, her worsening ability to converse, poor air movement, and new-onset lethargy). Sending her home would not be an option. This patient should be started on continuous nebulizer therapy and transferred to the ICU for close monitoring as soon as possible. Other treatment additions would include IV steroid and IV β-agonist therapies.

A. An ABG would help you determine if this patient was unable to oxygenate or ventilate (showing signs of tiring). This would be manifested even if a CO_2 level was normal, because it should NOT be normal in a patient that is breathing 30 times a minute and ventilating appropriately. The CO_2 would be a late sign that the patient was tiring and should worry you that this patient will need to be intubated soon.

B. This patient does need to be admitted, but observation on the floor would be inadequate. This patient has exhibited signs of impending respiratory decline with her lung exam, her decreasing ability to speak, and her worsening neurologic status.

C. Inhaled corticosteroid therapy is used in the treatment of mild persistent and moderate asthma. Use in the acute setting of status asthmaticus has not been shown to affect outcome.

D. In a patient with status asthmaticus, IV steroids should be started immediately and continued until asthma improves.

128. **A.** This patient likely has farmer's lung, the most common hypersensitivity pneumonitis. Symptoms are generally vague, presenting as malaise, fevers, and chills with associated cough. There may be some shortness of breath and even hemoptysis. Farmer's lung is caused by thermophilic actinomycetes that are present in moldy compost or hay.

B. Animal proteins can also be responsible for hypersensitivity pneumonitis. The most common form is bird-breeder's lung; bird droppings are responsible for the antigenic response. Other animal proteins that can cause this condition include rodent urine and shell dust.

C. Fungi can also cause hypersensitivity pneumonitis. Cheese worker's lung (*Penicillium* spp) and woodworker's lung (*Alternaria* spp) are other examples. Our patient gives no history of working with cheese or wood.

D. Work-related chemicals that can cause hypersensitivity pneumonitis include epoxy resin and trimellitic anhydride (plastic worker's lung). This patient gives no history of these exposures.

E. Arthropods, in particular the wheat weevil, *Sitophilus grainarius*, can cause hypersensitivity pneumonitis (miller's lung).

129. **D.** Avoidance of antigen exposure is difficult and can cause a financial burden on farmers with hypersensitivity pneumonitis. Reduction of antigenic burden can be difficult also; if compost or hay is wetted down before handling, the number of mobile actinomycetes is reduced. Avoidance of antigen is the primary treatment in hypersensitivity pneumonitis.

A. Inhaled β-agonist therapy has not been shown to help with farmer's lung. The major etiology of symptoms is diffuse inflammation of the lung parenchyma secondary to antigen exposure. A bronchodilator is not the first-line therapy.

B. High-dose IV steroids are not part of the initial treatment regiment for farmer's lung. Oral steroids have been studied and are used in patients with moderate symptoms.

C. Antibiotic therapy is not indicated as the mechanism for a patient's symptoms is inflammation of lung parenchyma secondary to antigen exposure and sensitization. Avoidance of antigen and treatment of inflammation are necessary therapies.

E. Oral steroids have been shown to result in some improvement in patients with moderate acute symptoms. In studies comparing steroids to antigen exposure removal, at 6 months patient symptoms were similar, suggesting that steroids can help in the acute phase.

130. **D.** The complement cascade is initiated when antibodies or immunoglobulins bind to an antigen. The cascade is composed of two parts, classical and alternative. The alternative differs from the classical in that it can be indirectly initiated by cell wall proteins. Hereditary angioedema is an autosomal dominant disorder. It is caused by a decrease in the C1-esterase inhibitory protein. This protein is responsible for the breakdown of the first part of the complement cascade to prevent excessive complement activation. With excessive complement activation, patients have increased bradykinin release, which increases vasopermeability. Patients are subject to asymmetric swelling of extremities, tongue, and larynx and do not have associated urticaria. Treatment is with androgens, which help increase levels of C1-esterase inhibitor. Fresh frozen plasma can be given to acutely replete C1 inhibitor. C1 inhibitor deficiency is different from mast cell-mediated forms of angioedema that respond to antihistamines. Itching is often a component of these forms of angioedema.

A. A deficiency of C5 through C9 results in increased infections with the *Neisseria* spp (meningococcal and gonococcal). Patients with recurrent disseminated gonococcal infections should be screened for terminal complement deficiency.

B. C3 deficiency leads to recurrent bacterial infections with encapsulated organisms. Patients present soon after birth.

C. C2 deficiency results in the development of lupus. It can also present in childhood with recurrence of pyogenic infections. It is the most common complement deficiency.

E. IgA deficiency is associated with recurrent sinopulmonary infections and celiac disease. It is not associated with intermittent edema of extremities, tongue, or larynx.

131. **A.** This patient is having an anaphylactic reaction, as evidenced by her respiratory distress, hives, and hypotension. IV epinephrine is first-line therapy in patients with anaphylaxis who present with hypotension and bronchospasm. It has been shown that delay of epinephrine therapy increases mortality.

B. IV steroids are used to prevent late-phase reactions in patients with IgE-mediated reactions. They do not work in the acute phase.

C. Antihistamines, including both H1 and H2 blockers, are used to prevent symptoms secondary to histamine release, such as hives and itching. It has been shown that it is more effective to use H1 and H2 blockers together. However, these will not help this patient's hypotension and respiratory distress.

D. Subcutaneous epinephrine is given if a patient has mild to moderate symptoms including urticaria and hives. It may be repeated every 15 to 20 minutes. If a patient develops respiratory distress or hypotension, IV epinephrine should be administered.

E. Inhaled β-agonists can be used in concert with IV epinephrine in patients suffering from respiratory distress due to anaphylaxis to help ease the bronchospasm. It will not help with the hypotension.

132. C. This patient likely has C2 deficiency, which is the most common complement deficiency in whites. It may present with lupus, or patients may have a history of recurrent pyogenic infections as children. The appropriate test is the total hemolytic complement activity test (CH50). This is an initial screen to determine whether there is a problem in the function of the complement cascade. Individual complement components can be measured after a positive test.

A. Serum immunoglobulins should be ordered in a person suspected to have a humoral immunity deficiency. Typically, these patients present with recurrent sinopulmonary infections with encapsulated organisms. Quantitative immunoglobulins can also be measured.

B. The NBT dye test measures the ability of phagocytes to generate oxygen radicals used in the killing of microbes. Tests of phagocytosis are ordered when a patient gives a history of recurrent skin and respiratory infections with bacteria and fungi.

D. Anti-nuclear antibodies are checked when an autoimmune disorder is suspected, not an immunodeficiency. It is important to remember, however, that some cases of lupus are due to complement deficiencies.

E. X-chromosome inactivation analysis is performed when Wiscott-Aldrich (recurrent infections, eczema, and diarrhea), severe X-linked combined immunodeficiency, or hyper-IgM syndromes are suspected.

133. C. This patient has classic findings of OA. It typically has a slow, progressive onset and is the result of chronic trauma. The joints that are typically affected are the weight-bearing joints (hip, knee, and spine) and the small joints in the hand (specifically the DIP and PIP joints). Patients with OA typically have less than 30 minutes of morning stiffness, whereas patients with RA have longer periods of stiffness. They also typically do not have other evidence of systemic illness (fevers, malaise, etc.). Changes seen on physical exam include bony deformities (nodules) at the DIP (Heberden's nodes) and PIP (Bouchard's nodes) joints. Crepitus is commonly felt on examination of the effected joint (especially the knee). Classic X-ray findings are osteophytes and narrowing of the joint space.

A. RA typically presents more acutely and has more systemic signs and symptoms associated with it. These include fevers, malaise, morning stiffness (lasting between 45 minutes and several hours), anorexia, and weight loss to name a few. The joints that are typically affected in RA include the PIP joints and the metacarpophalangeal joints—the DIP joints are spared. Although the knee is the most common single joint involved in RA, it tends to affect mostly the smaller joints in the body.

B. Although the majority of patients with SLE have joint involvement, it is rarely the only part of the body involved. Similarly to RA, patients with SLE typically have more systemic signs of illness (fever, malaise, etc.). In addition, they do not typically develop the bony changes or crepitus seen in patients with OA.

D. CPPD deposition disease is a crystalline arthropathy that can mimic many disease processes. It can present as pseudo-RA, pseudo-OA, or pseudo-ankylosing spondylitis, or can even be asymptomatic. It is most often referred to as pseudo-gout because of its acute presentation (fairly abrupt onset as a monoarticular arthritis with an exquisitely painful joint). CPPD disease usually involves the knee and spares the smaller joints. The onset of disease is not usually as rapid as gout. The joint examination during an acute attack of CPPD disease is similar to that of gout (single joint, very painful, may or may not have overlying redness and swelling). The radiologic feature that identifies CPPD disease is the presence of chondrocalcinosis (calcium deposition in the cartilage) seen on plain X-rays (usually of the knee).

E. Reactive arthritis, or acute gout attacks, typically present as an abrupt monoarticular arthritis often with overlying redness and swelling (can easily mimic a septic joint). The smaller joints are usually spared with the exception of the large toe (first metatarsophalangeal joint). Physical findings are discussed above. X-rays taken during an acute gout attack may well be normal. Patients with chronic gouty arthritis can develop tophi (uric acid deposits) and joint erosions on X-ray.

---

134. **D.** Weight reduction, aerobic exercise (e.g., swimming), and NSAIDs are the mainstay for initial treatment of osteoarthritis. Orthotics, braces, canes, and other assistive devices may be beneficial for some patients. Patients who fail more conservative medical treatment may benefit from intra-articular injections with glucocorticoids. However, oral steroid therapy is not indicated for the treatment of OA (remember, it's the result of trauma; it is not a systemic autoimmune process). Patients with more advanced disease affecting the hips or knees may be referred for consideration for arthroplasty.

A. Methotrexate is commonly used in the treatment of RA but has no indication for the treatment of OA.

B. Prednisone is commonly used in the treatment of autoimmune processes such as RA and SLE, but not for OA.

C. Allopurinol, a xanthine oxidase inhibitor, is used for the chronic treatment of gout to decrease the production of uric acid. It is of no benefit in the treatment of OA.

E. Colchicine is used in select patients for the treatment of an acute flare of gout.

---

135. **B.** This patient has a classic presentation of gout. Gout is a crystalline arthropathy that can present acutely and is often exquisitely painful. Although the joint that is most commonly affected is the first metatarsal-phalangeal (MTP) joint (referred to as podagra), the knee is often involved as well. The inflammation in the joint can be quite intense and resemble that of an infected joint (redness, warmth, swelling, pain with motion, etc.). During an initial attack, X-rays of the affected joint may appear normal. It is only after recurrent attacks or a long-standing history of gout do you see the bony changes (tophi, joint erosions). Synovial fluid analysis reveals clear fluid with monosodium urate crystals which have strong negative birefringence (i.e., they look like yellow needles when lined up with the polarizing light of the microscope). The remainder of the synovial fluid studies can mimic those of an infected joint (leukocytosis, etc.).

A. Septic arthritis needs to be excluded in any patient with the presentation of a monoarticular arthritis and a history of IV drug use. The presence of crystals in the synovial fluid helps us make the diagnosis of gout in this case. However, one has to maintain a high index of suspicion, because patients with underlying joint disease (gout, RA, etc.) are at higher risk for the development of septic arthritis (actually, both processes can be present at the same time).

C. CPPD deposition disease—also known as pseudogout—can have a very similar presentation. The joint distribution, onset of disease, and physical examination findings are very similar, but the joint aspirate and X-ray findings are different. Synovial fluid from a patient with CPPD disease reveals rhomboid crystals that are weakly positively birefringent. X-rays of the affected joint reveals chondrocalcinosis as discussed above.

D. Traumatic fracture is less likely given there was no history of trauma. Also, fractures often result in hemorrhagic effusions, which the patient did not have.

E. SLE is often accompanied by joint involvement, but it usually is not monoarticular. The joint involvement in SLE is more diffuse and symmetric (it can often mimic RA). In addition, if synovial fluid were obtained from a joint affected by SLE, it should not contain monosodium urate crystals.

136. **E.** Gouty arthritis results from the deposition of monosodium urate crystals in the joint space. Although patients with high serum uric acid levels are at increased risk of developing gout, it cannot be used to make the diagnosis of gout. Many patients have elevated serum uric acid levels but never develop gout. Even in patients who develop gout, it is not the degree of elevation of uric acid in the serum that precipitates deposition of the crystals into the joint space, but rather how fast the level of uric acid changes. That is why many patients with gout will have an acute flare of their disease when they are admitted to the hospital (where they receive IV fluids or diuretics that alter their uric acid levels). In addition, if a high uric acid level is abruptly lowered (e.g., with IV fluids), an acute gout flare may result even though the uric acid level may be measured as normal at that point.

A, B, C, D. See explanation for E.

137. **D.** Patients with gout develop hyperuricemia by two potential mechanisms. They either overproduce uric acid (idiopathic, leukemia, hemolytic anemia, G6PD, etc.) or undersecrete it (idiopathic, chronic renal disease, lead nephropathy, alcohol, diabetic ketoacidosis [DKA], drugs, etc.). The treatment of *acute* gout flares and *chronic* gout is different. For acute gout, indomethacin is the preferred treatment. Colchicine can also be used for acute gout, but it has more side effects, such as diarrhea, nausea, and abdominal pain. Both indomethacin and colchicine are contraindicated in renal insufficiency, in which case intra-articular or oral steroids may be used, or even narcotics alone, just to control pain. Notice that the treatment focus of the acute attack is to decrease inflammation, not to alter the uric acid level.

A. Drugs that are used to treat chronic gout focus on decreasing production (allo-purinol) or increasing renal excretion (probenecid). These drugs may precipitate an acute flare, because they change the uric acid level; therefore, they should *not* be initiated during an acute attack. Doing so may prolong the initial attack, which the patient will not be happy about.

B. IV nafcillin may be considered if septic arthritis were possible; however, this patient has gout.

C. Prednisone may be given during an acute attack of gout, but this should be considered only if the patient is unable to take oral NSAIDs or colchicine. Intra-articular steroids can also be given if the patient cannot be given other forms of treatment.

E. You would consider immobilizing an extremity if you were concerned about a fracture until you could further evaluate it. However, this patient's findings are not consistent with a fracture. Immobilization may offer comfort to the patient with an acute gout flare, but it will not halt the disease process.

138. **B.** This patient has AS. AS is one type of the seronegative spondylarthropathies that are immune mediated, usually involve the spine, and have asymmetric joint involvement. Reactive arthritis and psoriatic arthritis are other types of seronegative spondylarthropathies. Patients with AS, all of whom have symptomatic sacroiliitis, usually develop the disease during young adulthood. Men are more commonly afflicted with the disease (some argue that there is equal prevalence, but that women have a milder disease process and often miss detection). The pain associated with AS is always decreased with exercise. Common physical findings include decreased range of motion in the affected spine and tenderness over the sacroiliac joint. Patients with AS can also develop "sausage digits" (as can those with reactive and psoriatic arthritis). Classic radiographic findings include the formation of new bone on vertebral bodies near the annulus fibrosis (which gives the vertebral bodies the classic "shiny corner" or "window pane" appearance). In addition, syndesmophytes are commonly seen. These collections of bone growth between the vertebral bodies eventually cause the vertebrae to fuse and have the bamboo appearance. Sacroiliitis is commonly seen on plain X-rays, with occasional fusion of the sacroiliac joints.

A. Vertebral osteomyelitis should be considered in any patient with low back pain and a history of IV drug use. Patients with vertebral osteomyelitis may or may not have systemic signs of illness (fevers, malaise, etc.). Bacterial causes of osteomyelitis tend to produce a more abrupt and systemic illness. However, infections such as my-cobacterium (tuberculosis) or coccidioidomycosis can cause vertebral osteomyelitis with a more indolent course. One of the most reliable clinical signs of vertebral os-teomyelitis is pain with palpation over the affected spinous process (which the patient does not have).

C. Reactive arthritis is another type of seronegative spondylarthropathy. However, patients with reactive arthritis do not develop the X-ray findings like those seen in AS. Reactive arthritis is an acute arthritis that occurs as the result of an infection elsewhere in the body (e.g., *Chlamydia, Ureaplasma, Salmonella, Shigella, Yersinia, Klebsiella,* and *Campylobacter*). Reiter's syndrome is a term often used interchange-ably with reactive arthritis. Although both terms refer to a similar process, Reiter's syndrome should be used only when there is the triad of conjunctivitis, arthritis, and nongonococcal urethritis.

D. Although RA shares some of the features of AS (morning stiffness, improvement in symptoms with activity, etc.), it should be noted that RA typically does *not* affect the spine or sacroiliac joints.

E. IBD can result in enteropathic arthropathy, which are joint attacks related to flares of IBD, but not associated with sacroiliitis. These attacks typically involve only a few of the joints of the lower extremities and are followed by complete remission. Occasionally, these patients may develop erythema nodosum or pyoderma gangrenosum.

139. A. HLA-B27 is very common among patients with seronegative spondyloarthropathies. Approximately 90% of patients with AS will be positive for HLA-B27. Sixty percent to 80% of patients with Reiter's syndrome, 60% of patients with spondylitis with psoriasis or IBD, and 10% of the healthy population are HLA-B27 positive.

B. Blood culture is not likely to be positive, because this is not caused by an infectious process. Even in the presence of vertebral osteomyelitis, fewer than 50% of patients will have a positive blood culture.

C. Rheumatoid factor can be present in a variety of conditions, with the most obvious one being RA. Again, our patient has spinal involvement, which rarely happens in RA.

D. Anti-nuclear antibodies are present in approximately 10% of the normal population and are not useful in the diagnosis of AS. They are a very sensitive test for SLE (i.e., their absence makes SLE very unlikely), but not very specific (i.e., if they are positive, it doesn't confirm your diagnosis of SLE).

E. Stool guaiac positivity along with clinical features of IBD may support a diagnosis of enteropathic arthropathy; however, our patient had none of these. This type of arthropathy does not give the X-ray findings typically seen in AS.

140. E. The incidence of spinal cord injuries in patients with AS is ten times that of the normal population. Other important associated findings/complications include uveitis and aortitis. Approximately 30% of patients with AS will develop uveitis, which presents as unilateral pain, photophobia, and lacrimation. Fortunately, only approximately 3% of patients with AS will develop aortitis, which causes aortic insufficiency and CHF.

A, B, C, D. Nephritis, serositis, cerebritis, and cutaneous lesions are all complications of SLE, but are not associated with AS.

141. **C.** This patient has temporal headaches, jaw claudication, and amaurosis fugax, which are consistent with temporal arteritis. These patients often have scalp tenderness as well. Temporal arteritis, or giant cell arteritis, is one of the large vessel vasculitides. It is the result of the infiltration of the blood vessels arising from the aortic arch by multinucleated giant cells. This usually occurs in a patchy or segmental fashion along the artery. Patients with temporal arteritis are more often female, usually over 50 years of age, and with sedimentation rates >60. There is a strong association with polymyalgia rheumatica (30% to 50% of patients). Without treatment, approximately half of the patients with temporal arteritis will progress to develop ischemic optic neuropathy with blindness (unilateral).

A, E. The other two major types of large vessel vasculitis are Takayasu's arteritis and aortitis. Takayasu's arteritis typically affects younger women of Asian descent and results in "pulseless disease" (i.e., upper extremity claudication with arterial obstruction). They may or may not have associated Raynaud's syndrome. Aortitis is seen primarily in two conditions, ankylosing spondylitis and syphilis. Aortitis usually results in aortic insufficiency and CHF.

B. An embolic CVA could result in ischemic optic neuritis; however, it would not account for her jaw claudication. In addition, embolic CVAs are not usually accompanied by headaches.

D. SLE can be complicated by the development of cerebritis, which can result in a headache. However, there are often changes in mental status with cerebritis, and normally it is not accompanied by visual changes or jaw claudication.

142. **D.** This situation should be treated as a medical emergency, because the patient has started having visual involvement from her temporal arteritis. The patient should be immediately started on prednisone 60 mg per day. She should also have a biopsy of her temporal artery to confirm the diagnosis. The biopsy should be taken from a tender area of the artery, and a substantial piece should be obtained, because the disease can be patchy or segmental. Ideally, the biopsy is obtained before starting treatment; however, with visual field involvement, treatment should not be delayed to get a biopsy. The histologic changes seen in temporal arteritis take several weeks to resolve, so the biopsy can be delayed for a short time if necessary.

A. Initiating steroid therapy and obtaining arteriography may be reasonable if you were concerned about aortitis; however, this is not the typical presentation of aortitis.

B. Anti-nuclear antibodies are not helpful in the diagnosis of temporal arteritis.

C. Obtaining a CT scan of the brain and initiating anti-platelet therapy would be reasonable if there were concern for a thrombotic CVA.

E. The RPR can be useful in the diagnosis of syphilis, which can cause aortitis. However, this patient doesn't have findings consistent with aortitis. Penicillin is the treatment of choice for syphilis.

143. **D.** Felty's syndrome is composed of the triad of RA, splenomegaly, and neutropenia. It may also be associated with anemia and thrombocytopenia. It is most often seen in patients with high rheumatoid factor titers and subcutaneous rheumatoid nodules. Patients with significant neutropenia with Felty's syndrome may develop opportunistic infections. The treatment for Felty's syndrome is basically getting control of the RA with immunosuppressant medications such as methotrexate, glucocorticoids, and, sometimes, gold therapy. Methotrexate may cause neutropenia as a side effect, and it may be hard to tell if the neutropenia is due to methotrexate treatment or Felty's syndrome. Granulocyte colony stimulating factor (G-CSF) may be used to boost the white count in patients with recurrent infections. Splenectomy is reserved for patients with refractory disease.

A. It is important to understand the difference between uremia and azotemia. Azotemia is elevation of the blood urea nitrogen, usually seen in patients with renal insufficiency. Uremia is a constellation of symptoms experienced by a patient who is severely azotemic. The symptoms of uremia are nausea, vomiting, dysgeusia (which patients describe as a "metallic" taste in their mouths), encephalopathy, pericarditis, and pruritus. Neither uremia or azotemia is part of Felty's syndrome.

B. A prolonged partial thromboplastin time (aPTT) may indicate a lupus anticoagulant, a factor deficiency, or an inhibitor of the clotting cascade. It is not associated with Felty's syndrome.

C. Aspartate aminotransferase (AST) is an enzyme that may be released from hepatocytes or muscle cells when either of these tissues is injured. It is not elevated in Felty's syndrome.

E. Hyperbilirubinemia is either direct or indirect, meaning that the predominant portion of the elevated bilirubin is either conjugated or unconjugated, respectively. Direct hyperbilirubinemia can be a result of obstruction of bile anywhere along the outflow tract, either intrahepatically or extrahepatically. Direct hyperbilirubinemia is not a part of Felty's syndrome.

144. **B.** Besides Felty's syndrome, there are numerous other extra-articular manifestations of RA. These include pericarditis, myocarditis, amyloid renal disease, keratoconjunctivitis sicca (eye dryness), scleritis, episcleritis, pleuritis, severe bronchiolitis, pulmonary interstitial fibrosis, anemia of chronic disease, vasculitis (resembles polyarteritis nodosa), and rheumatoid nodules. Of these, the nodules, severe anemia, and Felty's syndrome occur more commonly in rheumatoid factor-positive patients. Echocardiographic evidence of pericardial effusion is seen in almost 50% of RA patients who have no clinical symptoms.

A. Peptic ulcer disease is not a complication of RA itself, but may be a complication of therapy with NSAIDs. The only GI symptoms seen in RA are xerostomia in patients with associated Sjögren's disease and intestinal ischemia in patients with associated vasculitis.

C. The anemia associated with RA is common and is a result of inflammatory cytokine-induced suppression of normal erythropoiesis resulting in anemia of chronic disease.

D. Glomerular disease resulting in proteinuria is uncommon in RA (whereas it is very common in SLE). Proteinuria may rarely occur in RA secondary to amyloid-induced renal disease, or it may more commonly occur secondary to drug therapy such as penicillamine or gold.

E. Pulmonary extra-articular manifestations of RA are common and include pleuritis with pleural effusion and interstitial fibrosis. Autopsy findings confirm histologic evidence of interstitial lung disease in most patients with RA, most of whom were never symptomatic. Spontaneous pneumothorax is an extremely rare complication.

145. | **B.** Methotrexate works by interfering with the cellular use of folic acid. The depletion of folic acid in rapidly dividing cells is thought to be responsible for the symptoms of stomatitis, alopecia, diarrhea, and bone marrow suppression. Patients with low baseline levels of folic acid before initiation of treatment with methotrexate may experience more of the toxicities of therapy. Furthermore, many studies have found that these side effects may be ameliorated by adding folate to the patient's medication regimen without significantly affecting the efficacy of therapy.

A. A rash may occur within days of each weekly dose of methotrexate and may clear before the next week's dose. Some patients may develop photosensitivity on the drug. These skin reactions are not significantly changed by the addition of folate therapy.

C. Interstitial lung disease from pneumonitis (that may progress to fibrosis) occurs in 3% to 5% of RA patients who are on methotrexate therapy, and is unrelated to folic acid depletion. A new cough in patients on methotrexate therapy needs to be completely evaluated for the possibility of lung-related toxicity. It can be confusing to know whether the patient's interstitial lung disease is related to the methotrexate or to the underlying RA. An open lung biopsy may be required to determine the etiology of the patient's disease.

D. Liver injury also may be seen with methotrexate therapy and is unrelated to folic acid depletion. Patients on methotrexate should have their liver enzymes followed regularly, and some advocate periodic liver biopsies to assess for possible liver damage.

E. Folate supplementation does not reverse or lessen the teratogenic effects of methotrexate therapy. Women of child-bearing age should not be given methotrexate therapy unless they completely understand the risks to an unborn fetus and comply with contraception. It is recommended that both men and women be off of methotrexate therapy for at least 3 months before conception to decrease the risks of teratogenicity.

146. **B.** The clinical presentation of aplastic anemia can include fatigue and pallor due to anemia, mucosal bleeding due to thrombocytopenia, and recurrent infections due to neutropenia. Peripheral blood counts will reveal pancytopenia with a normocytic anemia and poor reticulocyte count. Bone marrow aspirate shows all cell lines to be hypocellular with increased bone marrow fat cells. The causes of aplastic anemia include chemicals such as benzene and arsenic; drugs such as chloramphenicol and carbonic anhydrase inhibitors; and viral infections including cytomegalovirus, Epstein-Barr virus, and parvovirus. In many cases of aplastic anemia, a cause is never established. Ultimate cure is a bone marrow transplant.

A. Myelodysplastic syndromes have a clinical presentation that is similar to that of aplastic anemia, because both cause pancytopenia. However, myelodysplastic syndromes cause abnormal features of the cells that can be seen on the peripheral smear. In addition, bone marrow aspirate usually reveals hypercellularity with dysplasia of marrow precursor cells. Myelodysplastic syndromes are more common in elderly patients. The only definitive cure is chemotherapy followed by bone marrow transplant.

C. Paroxysmal nocturnal hemoglobinuria is also included in the differential of pancytopenia. It is an uncommon disease that includes chronic hemolytic anemia, pancytopenia, and thrombophilia. Cells are predisposed to lysis because of a defective membrane protein.

D. Chronic myelogenous leukemia can cause anemia; however, leukocyte count is typically elevated. Acute leukemias are more likely to cause pancytopenia.

E. Severe folate deficiency can cause pancytopenia. The anemia caused by folate deficiency is megaloblastic with MCV values above 100 fL. Hypersegmented neutrophils should also be seen on peripheral blood smear with folate deficiency.

147. **C.** Phlebotomy is the treatment of choice for polycythemia vera. The treatment consists of phlebotomy once or twice weekly until the patient is iron deficient and hemoglobin is <14 g/dL. Hydroxyurea can also be used in conjunction with phlebotomy to control blood counts.

A. A low-to-normal serum erythropoietin level is consistent with polycythemia vera. An elevated level can be seen in secondary erthyrocytosis due to pulmonary disease, smoking, or sleep apnea.

B. RBC mass studies can be useful in confirming the diagnosis of polycythemia vera. RBC mass is elevated in polycythemia vera, but not in other myeloproliferative disorders. It cannot distinguish polycythemia vera from secondary erythrocytosis, because RBC mass can be elevated in both.

D. Splenomegaly is a common physical exam finding in polycythemia vera occurring in nearly 70% of patients. It does not necessarily indicate an underlying leukemia. Patients with polycythemia vera do have a 2% to 5% lifetime risk of leukemic transformation, but splenomegaly is not a specific physical finding to indicate this transformation.

E. Fifty percent to 60% of patients have an elevated platelet count. Forty percent to 50% of patients have an elevated WBC count.

148. **D.** The smear in Figure 148 shows a macrocytic anemia. Patients with Crohn's disease often have inflammation of the distal ileum where B_{12} is absorbed, leading to the deficiency. A B_{12} level can be obtained to confirm the diagnosis.

A. Patients with Crohn's disease can have iron-deficiency anemia due to iron malabsorption with duodenal involvement, or due to chronic GI bleeding. However, iron deficiency causes a microcytic anemia, and Figure 148 shows a macrocytic anemia.

B. Anemia secondary to blood loss, if acute, is typically normocytic. If the blood loss is chronic, a microcytic anemia can be seen due to iron deficiency. This patient has a macrocytic anemia.

C. Anemia of chronic disease can be seen in Crohn's disease, but it will be a microcytic or normocytic anemia.

E. Folate deficiency is a macrocytic anemia. However, folate deficiency is not typically seen in patients with Crohn's disease.

149. **C.** Iron-deficiency anemia is treated most commonly with ferrous sulfate. Reticulocyte count can be expected to increase within 7 to 10 days after starting iron therapy. Hemoglobin levels increase over the first month of treatment with an increase of 2 g/dL being considered an adequate response to treatment. It is important, however, to determine whether a patient has iron deficiency before putting them on iron supplements.

A. In iron-deficiency anemia, iron studies show low iron, high total iron binding capacity, and low ferritin. The profile shown of low iron, low total iron binding capacity, and high ferritin is consistent with anemia of chronic disease.

B. The most common cause of iron-deficiency anemia is blood loss either from the GI tract or from menstrual bleeding. Intake of iron is adequate for most people, with the exception of pregnant women and toddlers.

D. Pica (which means eating "non-nutritive" substances) occurs in over 50% of patients with untreated iron-deficiency anemia. The word specific for ice craving is "pagophagia."

E. Ferritin is an acute phase reactant and is affected by acute illness, infectious processes, and chronic diseases. However, ferritin is also the best predictor of iron stores. Even in the face of chronic illness or inflammatory disease, a ferritin greater than 100 mg/L rules out an iron deficiency state.

150. **B.** This patient has a history and peripheral smear that indicates hereditary spherocytosis. This is the most common hemolytic anemia due to an RBC membrane defect. Inheritance is autosomal dominant. Patients with a milder form can present into early adulthood with anemia and cholelithiasis. Typical laboratory findings include anemia with elevated reticulocyte count. MCV is usually not helpful, but the mean corpuscular hemoglobin concentration (MCHC), and red cell distribution width (RDW) can be elevated. Peripheral smear will show spherocytes with hemolytic cell fragments as depicted in Figure 150. Diagnosis should be confirmed with the osmotic fragility test. In this test, RBCs are placed in progressively more dilute saline solutions. Spherocytes hemolyze at hypotonic concentrations at which normal cells survive.

A. Bone marrow biopsy is not necessary. The diagnosis can be obtained through clinical history, peripheral smear, and osmotic fragility testing.

C. History and peripheral smear are not consistent with G6PD deficiency. There is no history of a new medication, infection, or other offending agent in this patient.

D. Splenectomy may be indicated in this patient for future treatment, but should not be done before diagnosis is confirmed. It is indicated in patients with moderate to severe anemia who require multiple transfusion therapies. The risk of splenectomy is later development of infection and sepsis with encapsulated organisms. All patients who receive a splenectomy should receive pneumococcal, haemophilus, and meningococcal vaccines a few weeks before surgery.

E. IgG and IgM autoantibody levels could be obtained if immune-mediated hemolytic anemia were suspected. History and peripheral smear do not suggest this diagnosis.

Questions

151. You are seeing a new patient in your clinic who comes to establish care. He is a 24-year-old man from the Mediterranean region with a history of anemia since childhood. You consider the possibility of a hemolytic anemia. Which of the following statements is true regarding hemolytic anemia?

A. Hemolytic anemia occurs only when there is destruction of the erythrocyte by an antibody

B. Direct bilirubin and haptoglobin levels are elevated

C. Pyruvate kinase deficiency is the most common cause of enzyme deficiency hemolysis in RBCs

D. IgG antibodies are associated with cold autoimmune hemolytic anemia

E. Glucose 6-phosphate dehydrogenase (G6PD) deficiency is an X-linked disorder that induces hemolysis after exposure to oxidant drugs

152. A 25-year-old black man with sickle cell anemia presents with 1 day of chest pain, cough, and fever. Physical examination is remarkable for tachypnea with oxygen saturations of 88% on room air, tachycardia, and diminished breath sounds in the right lower lobe. A chest X-ray reveals a new infiltrate in the right lower lobe. Which of the following is the most appropriate next step in the management of acute chest syndrome?

A. Start IV heparin protocol

B. Begin ceftriaxone and azithromycin

C. Exchange transfusion

D. Limited supplemental oxygen to keep paO_2 at 70

E. Aggressive IV fluid hydration

153. A 28-year-old previously healthy woman presents with petechiae and epistaxis for the last 2 weeks. She denies fatigue, fever, weight loss, or any other associated symptoms. She takes no medications and has no significant past medical history. Physical examination is notable for scattered petechiae over the lower and upper extremities. No hepatosplenomegaly or mucous membrane lesions are noted. Labs are as follows: WBCs 8200/μL; differential normal; hemoglobin 15.4 g/dL; hematocrit 36%; platelets 14,000/μL; PT 12.1 seconds; PTT 21 seconds; bleeding time 2 minutes. The most likely diagnosis is:

A. Drug-induced thrombocytopenia

B. Acute autoimmune thrombocytopenia

C. Von Willebrand's disease

D. Hemophilia A

E. Hypersplenism

The response options for items 154 through 157 are the same. You will be required to select one answer for each item in the set.

A. Von Willebrand's disease

B. Hemophilia A

C. Vitamin K deficiency

D. Disseminated intravascular coagulation (DIC)

E. Hemophilia B

For each of the laboratory results, select the most likely clinical syndrome.

154. Prolonged prothrombin time (PT) that corrects when mixed with normal plasma; decreased factor VII; and prolonged PTT if severe

155. Slightly elevated activated partial thromboplastin time (aPTT); prolonged bleeding time; low factor VIII

156. Prolonged PTT; prolonged PT; low fibrinogen

157. Prolonged PTT; normal bleeding time; low factor VIII

End of set

---

158. A 28-year-old woman with history of SLE presents with shortness of breath and pleuritic chest pain that was acute in onset 4 hours ago. She has had two pregnancies complicated by spontaneous abortions in the first trimester. On physical examination she is tachypneic and tachycardic, and oxygen saturations are 85% on room air. Pulmonary examination reveals no focal crackles, wheezes, or other abnormalities. Arterial blood gas shows a respiratory alkalosis with hypoxia. Which of the following would be the most likely laboratory finding in this patient?

A. No correction of prolonged aPTT with addition of normal patient plasma serum
B. Normal aPTT time
C. Elevated platelet count
D. Prolonged PT
E. Negative anti-cardiolipin antibody

159. A 32-year-old white man with no significant past medical history presents with a 3-day history of right calf swelling and warmth. He completed a cross-country car trip 2 days ago. He denies shortness of breath, chest pain, or any other symptoms. The patient's father has a history of recurrent deep venous thrombosis (DVT) with pulmonary embolism. Physical examination is normal except for significant swelling of the right calf with a palpable cord. The patient is admitted, and an evaluation for hypercoagulable state is begun. The most likely underlying disorder in this patient would be:

A. Protein C deficiency
B. Antithrombin deficiency
C. Anti-phospholipid syndrome
D. Malignancy
E. Factor V Leiden defect

160. A 63-year-old woman presents to your office for preoperative evaluation for a total knee replacement. Her past medical history is significant only for osteoarthritis for which she takes nonsteroidal anti-inflammatory drugs (NSAIDs). She is concerned about the possibility of a blood transfusion either during the surgery or during the postoperative period. She asks about the risks of transfusion therapy. Which of the following is a true statement regarding transfusion therapy?

A. The patient should be transfused for a hemoglobin of 10 g/dL
B. Acute hemolytic transfusion reactions occur primarily in patients who have had many transfusions
C. HIV is the most common viral infection that can be acquired from a transfusion
D. The risk of acquiring hepatitis C from a blood transfusion is approximately 1:100,000 units of blood transfused
E. Delayed transfusion reaction is usually due to ABO incompatibility

---

The next two questions (items 161 and 162) correspond to the following vignette.

A 45-year-old white woman comes to your office for a new patient visit. She denies any current concerns or complaints. She has no past medical history except for obesity. She has a family history of diabetes, type II. She denies tobacco use and IV drug use. She drinks socially once or twice per month. She is interested in starting an exercise regimen and diet. On exam the patient is afebrile, pulse is 90, respiratory rate 18, blood pressure 125/76, and BMI 31. In general she is obese, in no acute distress. Exam is essentially within normal limits with the exception of the following skin findings seen in Figure 161.

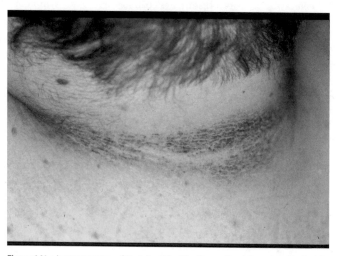

Figure 161 • Image courtesy of Dr. Robert Raschke, Banner Good Samaritan Medical Center, Phoenix, Arizona

161. This skin finding is called:

A. Acanthosis nigricans
B. Necrobiosis lipoidica
C. Granuloma annulare
D. Tinea corporis
E. Carotenodermia

162. You are concerned that this patient may have type II diabetes. Which of the following values confirms the diagnosis of diabetes?

A. A random plasma glucose >190 mg/dL
B. A fasting plasma glucose >126 mg/dL
C. A 2-hour plasma glucose concentration >140 mg/dL during an oral glucose tolerance test
D. A hemoglobin A1C >7.0
E. Ketosis and an anion gap acidosis

End of set

163. A 32-year-old white woman presents to your office with amenorrhea. She states she is not sexually active. She has had regular periods for most of her life until recently. She also notes the recent onset of headaches that are frontal and constant in nature. She does not note any visual changes. Physical exam is essentially normal with the exception of galactorrhea. A pregnancy test is negative and prolactin level is 500 ng/mL. The next diagnostic step in this patient is:

A. CT of the brain
B. MRI of the brain
C. Skull films
D. Review of the patient's medication list
E. A bromocriptine trial

164. A 24-year-old white woman presents to your office with symptoms of weight loss and diarrhea and complaints of sweating. These symptoms have progressed for approximately 1 month. She denies any past medical history. She also denies any tobacco, alcohol, or drug use. She currently takes no medications or herbs and family history is noncontributory. On physical exam the patient is afebrile, thin appearing with stable vital signs. HEENT is notable for lid lag bilaterally, and neck exam is notable for thyromegaly without bruit or obvious nodule. Heart and lung exam are within normal limits. Neurologic exam is significant for hyperreflexia throughout. Skin is noted to be warm with fine hair throughout. The most likely cause of this patient's symptoms is:

A. Subacute thyroiditis
B. Toxic adenoma
C. Addison's disease
D. Hashimoto's thyroiditis
E. Graves' disease

165. A 19-year-old white man is brought to your office by his parents. They are concerned that he has become more distant. He has lost 20 pounds in the last 4 months and has intermittent abdominal pain and nausea. He has also complained of increasing fatigue. He denies any past medical problems, tobacco, alcohol, or drug use. On physical exam, his heart rate is 110, respiratory rate 18, blood pressure 90/60, and oxygen saturations are 99 percent on room air. On exam he appears thin and withdrawn. His lungs are clear, and his heart is tachycardic without murmurs. His abdomen is soft without hepatosplenomegaly. He appears slightly tanned, especially in his palmar creases. You order basic labs that reveal the following: WBC 6000/μL; eosinophils 8%; hemoglobin 14 g/dL; sodium 130 mEq/dL; potassium 5.8 mEq/dL; chloride 107 mEq/dL; bicarbonate 24 mEq/L; BUN 18 mg/dL; creatinine 0.8 mg/dL; glucose 68 mg/dL. What is the most likely diagnosis?

A. Hyperthyroidism
B. Hypothyroidism
C. Primary hypoadrenalism
D. Secondary hypoadrenalism
E. Hyperaldosteronism

166. A 35-year-old white woman presents to your office with complaints of irregular menses. She started menstruating at age 15. Her periods have always been irregular, occurring every 28 to 50 days. She is currently trying to get pregnant and has been trying for more than 3 years. She is on phenobarbital for a seizure disorder. She denies any illicit drug, alcohol, or tobacco use. Vital signs are within normal limits. Her BMI is 28. Physical exam is notable for dark hair on her upper lips, arms, and abdomen. She has mild acne on her face and her upper back. Initial CBC is normal and pregnancy test is negative. TSH is 3.5 mU/L and free T4 is normal. The most likely cause of her hirsutism is:

A. Idiopathic hirsutism
B. Polycystic ovarian syndrome
C. Pituitary neoplasm
D. Phenobarbital
E. Hypothyroidism

167. A 75-year-old Hispanic man was recently seen in the ED for complaints of fatigue, weight loss of 15 pounds in 6 months, and cough. He has brought the results of basic labs taken at that time to your office and wants you to interpret the results. The patient has a past medical history significant for hypertension on a β-blocker and a smoking history of one pack per day for 40 years. Vitals are within normal limits with the exception of a respiratory rate of 24 and saturations of 90% on room air. Exam is significant for a thin man in no acute distress. Lung exam is significant for decreased breath sounds at the left lung base. The rest of his exam is essentially normal. The labs values are: Sodium 140 mEq/dL; potassium 4.6 mEq/dL; chloride 105 mEq/dL; bicarbonate 23 mEq/L; BUN 27 mg/dL; creatinine 1.1 mg/dL; glucose 80 mg/dL; calcium 12.5 mg/dL. The most likely etiology for this man's laboratory abnormality is:

A. Parathyroid adenoma
B. Sarcoidosis
C. Squamous cell lung carcinoma
D. β-blocker
E. Thyrotoxicosis

168. A 24-year-old white woman presents to your office with complaints of palpitations, shaking hands, and sweatiness. She states the symptoms started about 1 hour ago. You quickly review her chart and see that she has a medical history significant for depression and one suicide attempt 5 years ago. She denies any ingestions, drug, alcohol, or tobacco use. Her family history is significant for depression and type I diabetes in a 14-year-old sister. Her vital signs are within normal limits, but she is pale and diaphoretic. You check a glucose level and it is 30 mg/dL. As you replete her glucose stores, you order some lab tests. Which would be the most helpful in determining the etiology of her hypoglycemia?

A. Insulin level
B. C-peptide level
C. Sulfonylurea level
D. Liver enzyme tests (AST and ALT)
E. Thyroid function tests

169. A 36-year-old white woman comes to your office with her husband. He states that for the last few days she has been complaining of diffuse abdominal pain and bone pain. Today he noted that she was acting a bit confused. She has a past medical history significant for hypertension for which she takes a thiazide diuretic. This has never happened before, and she denies any alcohol, drug, or tobacco use. She has not had any fevers or chills, nausea, vomiting, or diarrhea. He thinks she has been constipated lately. On exam, temperature is 98.8°F (37.1°C), heart rate 80, respiratory rate 16, blood pressure 140/80, and oxygen saturations 99% on room air. Abdominal exam is significant for mild left lower quadrant pain to deep palpation. On neurologic exam, cranial nerves II through XII are intact, and muscle strength and sensorium are intact. Deep tendon reflexes are diminished throughout. You order basic labs, which reveal the following: CBC normal; sodium 140 mEq/L; potassium 4.6 mEq/L; chloride 108 mEq/L; bicarbonate 24 mEq/L; BUN 28 mg/dL; creatinine 0.8 mg/dL; glucose 90 mg/dL; calcium 13.0 mg/dL. The next step in the treatment of this patient is:

A. Glucocorticoid
B. Furosemide
C. Bisphosphonate
D. Calcitonin
E. Normal saline bolus

170. A 55-year-old white man comes to your office for routine check-up. He currently has no complaints. He has well-controlled hypertension on a β-blocker and a history of gout controlled with NSAIDs. His exam is essentially within normal limits. You note that he has not had a cholesterol level checked in the last 5 years. The fasting lipid panel reveals: LDL 116 mg/dL; HDL 50 mg/dL; triglycerides 600 mg/dL. You decide to start him on a fibrate. The mechanism by which this medication works is:

A. Reduces secretion of very low density lipoprotein (VLDL), increases stimulation of lipoprotein lipase
B. Reduces intrahepatic cholesterol, leading to increases in LDL receptor turnover
C. Inhibits production of VLDL, reduces transfer of HDL to VLDL
D. Binds bile acids in the intestine, thus lowering the cholesterol pool
E. Impairs dietary cholesterol absorption at the intestinal brush border

The response options for items 171 through 175 are the same. You will be required to select one answer for each item in the set.

    A. Elevated calcium, low phosphate, elevated parathyroid hormone (PTH)
    B. Elevated calcium, variable phosphate, low PTH
    C. Low calcium, elevated phosphate, low PTH
    D. Low calcium, elevated phosphate, elevated PTH
    E. Low or normal calcium, low phosphate, elevated PTH

For each disease state, select the most appropriate laboratory findings.

171. Vitamin D deficiency

172. Malignancy

173. Hypoparathyroidism

174. Pseudohypoparathyroidism

175. Hyperparathyroidism

End of set

176. A 65-year-old Hispanic man comes to your office with concerns regarding his sexual function. He states that he has had no difficulty obtaining erections until the last couple of months. He denies any recent psychosocial stressors and tells you that he has occasionally awakened with an erection during this time period. He has a past medical history significant for hypertension and is taking a thiazide diuretic. His physical exam is essentially within normal limits, including normal testicular size and firmness and a positive cremasteric reflex. What is the most likely cause of his erectile dysfunction?

    A. Neurogenic
    B. Vascular
    C. Medication induced
    D. Depression
    E. Hypogonadism

The response options for items 177 through 180 are the same. You will be required to select one answer for each item in the set.

    A. Anti-phospholipid antibody syndrome
    B. DIC
    C. Von Willebrand's disease
    D. Hemophilia A
    E. Hemophilia B

For each clinical scenario, select the most appropriate laboratory results.

177. A 36-year-old gravida 2 para 0 woman presents with new DVT. Laboratories show thrombocytopenia and an elevated PTT that does not correct when mixed with normal plasma. PT is normal.

178. A 17-year-old man presents with right knee hemarthrosis. Laboratories show prolonged PTT, normal PT, normal bleeding time, and low factor IX.

179. A 28-year-old woman presents with menorrhagia and easy bruising. Laboratories show slightly elevated aPTT, prolonged bleeding time, and low factor VIII.

180. A 76-year-old man is admitted to the intensive care unit for urosepsis. Laboratories show prolonged PTT, prolonged PT, decreased platelets, and low fibrinogen.

End of set

The response options for items 181 through 185 are the same. You will be required to select one answer for each item in the set.

A. Multiple myeloma
B. Primary hyperparathyroidism
C. Familial hypocalciuric hypercalcemia
D. Sarcoidosis
E. Squamous cell carcinoma

For each disease, select the associated mechanism of hypercalcemia.

181. Excessive secretion of PTH by a parathyroid adenoma or by parathyroid hyperplasia

182. Excessive renal tubular absorption of calcium and magnesium

183. Parathyroid hormone-related peptide (PTH-rP) production

184. Elevated concentrations of 1,25-dihydroxyvitamin D secondary to the excessive conversion of 25-hydroxyvitamin D to 1,25-dihydroxyvitamin D (the active metabolite)

185. Cytokine-mediated activation of osteoclasts, which resorb bone

End of set

The response options for items 186 through 190 are the same. You will be required to select one answer for each item in the set.

A. Ginkgo biloba
B. Echinacea
C. Ginseng
D. Saw palmetto
E. St. John's wort

For each disorder, select the most commonly used herbal medication.

186. Benign prostatic hypertrophy (BPH)

187. Depression

188. Dementia

189. Respiratory infections

190. Fatigue

End of set

The response options for items 191 through 193 are the same. You will be required to select one answer for each item in the set.

    A. Initiate drug therapy
    B. Initiate diet therapy
    C. No therapy

For each clinical scenario, select the appropriate management. Each answer may be used more than once.

191. A 56-year-old white man with a past medical history significant for hypertension comes to your office for a routine follow-up. His blood pressure is fairly well controlled. Exam is essentially within normal limits. You order basic labs and note an LDL of 176 mg/dL.

192. A 45-year-old Hispanic woman comes to your office for a well woman exam. She has no significant past medical history. She is active and denies any tobacco, alcohol, or drug use. Her mother has been told she has elevated cholesterol, and the patient would like to be checked. Her LDL is 170 mg/dL.

193. A 65-year-old white woman with a recent myocardial infarction comes to your office for a post-hospitalization checkup. Her current medications include a β-blocker, an angiotensin-converting enzyme (ACE) inhibitor, and aspirin. A check of her cholesterol reveals an LDL of 130 mg/dL.

End of set

The response options for items 194 through 199 are the same. You will be required to select one answer for each item in the set.

    A. Perifollicular purpura
    B. Perifollicular hyperkeratosis
    C. Hypopigmented macules and patches on flexural skin areas
    D. Alopecia
    E. Erythema, edema, blisters, and bullae of the dorsa of the hands
    F. Angular stomatitis
    G. Seborrhea

For each vitamin deficiency, select the most likely skin finding.

194. Vitamin A

195. Vitamin B$_3$ (niacin)

196. Vitamin B$_2$ (riboflavin)

197. Vitamin B$_{12}$ (cyanocobalamin)

198. Vitamin C

199. Vitamin B$_6$ (pyridoxine)

End of set

200. A 50-year-old Hispanic man with a history of hypertension comes to your office as a new patient. He has no complaints, but his family history is significant for several members with type II diabetes mellitus, and he is concerned that he also might develop the disease. On physical exam, his blood pressure is 140/90 and other vital signs are within normal limits. His BMI is 32 and you note a velvety dark pigment on the back of his neck and his axillary regions. His fasting glucose is 149 and 151 on two separate evaluations. What is the appropriate management for this patient with newly diagnosed diabetes?

    A. Diet and exercise therapy alone
    B. Diet and exercise, begin metformin as monotherapy
    C. Diet and exercise, begin a sulfonylurea as monotherapy
    D. Diet and exercise, begin long-acting lantus insulin as monotherapy
    E. Confirm the diagnosis with an elevated hemoglobin A1C

Answers and Explanations

FOUR

Answer Key

151. E	168. B	185. A
152. B	169. E	186. D
153. B	170. A	187. E
154. C	171. E	188. A
155. A	172. B	189. B
156. D	173. C	190. C
157. B	174. D	191. A
158. A	175. A	192. B
159. E	176. C	193. A
160. D	177. A	194. B
161. A	178. E	195. E
162. B	179. C	196. F
163. B	180. B	197. C
164. E	181. B	198. A
165. C	182. C	199. G
166. B	183. E	200. B
167. C	184. D	

151. **E.** G6PD deficiency is the most common enzymatic deficiency in RBCs. It can induce a hemolytic anemia after exposure to oxidant drugs such as sulfa, dapsone, and primaquine. Hemolysis can also be induced by infection and other agents, including fava beans.

A. Hemolytic anemia can be caused by membrane defects, enzyme abnormalities, hemoglobinopathies, immune or autoimmune processes, or drugs.

B. Laboratory findings in hemolytic anemia include an elevated reticulocyte count, an elevated indirect bilirubin, an elevated lactate dehydrogenase level, and a *decreased* haptoglobin.

C. G6PD deficiency is the most common RBC enzymatic defect.

D. IgM antibodies are associated with cold autoimmune hemolytic anemia. IgG antibodies are associated with warm autoimmune hemolytic anemia. You can remember this as follows: When I am *warm*, I want a *glass* of iced tea (Warm: IgG); When I am *cold*, I want a *mug* of hot cocoa (Cold: IgM). In both disorders, 50% of the patients have an underlying disorder such as AIDS, systemic lupus erythematosus (SLE), or inflammatory bowel disease.

152. **B.** The cause of acute chest syndrome is not fully known. Both infection and infarction have been indicated as possible causes. Therefore, it is appropriate to treat the patient for both community-acquired organisms and atypical pneumonias.

A. Anticoagulation therapy should be started only if there is a documented thromboembolic event.

C. Exchange transfusion is indicated in acute chest syndrome if there are progressive infiltrates on chest X-ray or progressive hypoxia.

D. Supplemental oxygen is necessary to prevent further sickling. PaO_2 should be maintained above 70, and brought to 100 if possible.

E. IV fluid hydration is important in the management of acute chest syndrome, but should be monitored closely. Fluid hydration that is too aggressive can lead to pulmonary edema.

153. **B.** This patient has a low platelet count with no other associated cytopenias. There is no history of medications or other underlying illnesses. Autoimmune thrombocytopenia is a diagnosis of exclusion. It is due to anti-platelet antibodies directed against membrane proteins. The process can be self-limited, or it can reoccur and become chronic. Treatment includes steroids, IV immune globulin (IVIG), and possible splenectomy if other treatments fail.

A. Drug-induced thrombocytopenia is due to a medication that causes destruction of platelets. Heparin is the most well-known offending drug. It causes platelet destruction by heparin-dependent antibodies that act against platelets.

C. Von Willebrand's disease is an autosomal-dominant inherited disorder of hemostasis. It affects platelet function, but does not affect platelet count.

D. Hemophilia A is an X-linked inherited bleeding disorder. It does not affect platelet count. Partial thromboplastin time is prolonged. Patients usually present with prolonged bleeding, hematomas, or hemarthrosis.

E. Hypersplenism can cause a decreased platelet count, leading to petechiae. This patient does not have a palpable spleen on exam and has no underlying diagnosis that would account for an enlarged spleen.

154.	**C.** Vitamin K deficiency initially prolongs PT with decreased factor VII levels. As other factors begin to decrease, the PTT will also prolong. Vitamin K-dependent factors include factors II, VII, IX, and X; protein C; and protein S. Replacement with vitamin K will correct the coagulopathy.

155.	**A.** Von Willebrand's disease is the most common inherited bleeding disorder. Patients usually have easy bruising, nosebleeds, menorrhagia, or prolonged bleeding with trauma. Von Willebrand factor plays a critical role in platelet function and is also a carrier protein for factor VIII. Defective von Willebrand factor can therefore decrease factor VIII and prolong PTT.

156.	**D.** DIC is triggered by systemic illness and can be a catastrophic hematologic event. Possible associations with DIC include sepsis, trauma, malignancy, and burns. Initially, fibrinogen and platelets are consumed in clot formation. This is later followed by hemorrhage as the clots are degraded by fibrinolysis.

157.	**B.** Hemophilia A is an X-linked inherited bleeding disorder. Patients usually present with prolonged bleeding, hematomas, or hemarthrosis. In hemophilia A, factor VIII is deficient.

E. Hemophilia B is due to a factor IX deficiency. (It is also called "Christmas disease.") Patients present with varying degrees of bleeding secondary to the deficient factor IX. This is also an X-linked recessive disease like hemophilia A.

158.	**A.** This patient has anti-phospholipid antibody syndrome. Patients with this syndrome have antibodies directed toward certain phospholipid-bound plasma proteins that are involved in the coagulation pathway. Patients are predisposed to recurrent arterial and venous clot formation as well as fetal loss. This syndrome is more commonly seen in patients with autoimmune syndromes, but can also be associated with malignancies, infections, and some drugs. Laboratory testing includes lupus anticoagulant. The patient's serum is mixed with normal patient serum to see if the aPTT corrects. If no correction is seen, this indicates that there is an "inhibitor" present, which in this patient is most likely a lupus anticoagulant.

B. Activated PTT can be normal in anti-phospholipid antibody syndrome, but typically is elevated.

C. Thrombocytopenia is associated with this syndrome not thrombocytosis.

D. PT is not affected by the lupus anticoagulant.

E. Anti-cardiolipin is one of the anti-phospholipid antibodies and can be positive in this syndrome. It is detected by enzyme-linked immunosorbent assay (ELISA).

159. E. Factor V Leiden defect is the most common inherited hypercoagulable state accounting for nearly 50% of inherited thrombophilic disorders. Estimated prevalence of the defect is 2% to 5%, with whites having the highest prevalence. The risk of venous thrombosis in patients who are heterozygous for this defect is approximately seven times that of persons without the defect. Several factors should alert the clinician to an underlying defect, including family history of thrombosis, age of first thrombotic event <50, and recurrent thrombotic events.

A. Protein C deficiency is less common, with a prevalence of less than 1%. Protein C, once activated, breaks down factors V and VIII. This deficiency is associated with a high incidence of thrombosis, even among patients who are heterozygous. Most patients present in their 20s or 30s with a venous thromboembolism.

B. Antithrombin inactivates procoagulant factors including factors II, IX, and X. Initial presentation with thrombosis typically occurs before age 50. This defect also has a prevalence of less than 1%.

C. Anti-phospholipid antibodies occur in 2% to 5% of otherwise healthy people, but are most frequent in patients with autoimmune disorders such as SLE. Patients with this syndrome are at risk for both venous and arterial thromboembolisms.

D. Malignancy is a risk factor for hypercoagulable state; however, this patient has no history to suggest this as an underlying diagnosis.

160. D. Hepatitis C is the second most common viral infection that can be acquired from blood transfusion. Hepatitis B is the most common with a risk of 1 : 60,000 units transfused. Although all blood is screened for infection, current screening methods do not detect early stages or some subclinical infections.

A. There is no evidence to support transfusion of an asymptomatic patient with no underlying cardiovascular disease based solely on the hemoglobin level.

B. Acute hemolytic transfusion reactions are serious and life-threatening, and can occur in any patient receiving a blood transfusion. Acute hemolytic transfusion reactions are due to ABO incompatibility. Symptoms include fever and back pain with development of renal failure.

C. Hepatitis B and C have a higher transmission rate than HIV. The risk of acquiring HIV from a blood transfusion is 1 : 500,000 units transfused.

E. Delayed transfusion reactions are seen in patients who have developed autoantibodies due to prior transfusion or pregnancy. Rh, Kidd, Duffy, and Kell are the typical antigens to which the antibodies are directed. Onset of delayed transfusion reaction can occur by 5 to 10 days after transfusion and manifests with fever, jaundice, and anemia due to extravascular hemolysis.

161. **A.** Acanthosis nigricans is a common manifestation of insulin resistance, often seen in patients with type II diabetes. It is a nonspecific skin reaction that presents with symmetric brown thickening of the skin. Acanthosis can develop a warty-like appearance and is typically found in the axilla, neck flexures, and groin. It is also seen in syndromes of excess steroid, in obesity, and in other endocrine disorders.

B. Necrobiosis lipoidica is unknown in its origin but approximately 50% of patients with this condition have diabetes. It usually appears before onset of diabetes in the third or fourth decade in women. Lesions are oval, violaceous patches that have a red, slowly expanding border. The central portion of the lesion is brown with telangiectasias.

C. Granuloma annulare is a ring-shaped, firm, flesh-colored papule. It is usually found on the lateral and dorsal portions of the hands and feet. Isolated lesions have no association with diabetes, but disseminated lesions do. These lesions usually spontaneously involute.

D. Tinea corporis is a fungal infection of the skin. Diabetics do have a predisposition to fungal infections, but more often in the form of thrush or vaginal candidiasis.

E. Carotenodermia is the yellowing of skin seen in diabetes and hypothyroidism.

162. **B.** Diagnostic criteria for diabetes include any one of the following: 1) a fasting blood sugar $\geq$126 mg/dL on two separate occasions; 2) a random blood sugar $\geq$200 mg/dL in a patient with symptoms of diabetes such as polyuria, polydipsia, and weight loss; and 3) a 2-hour plasma glucose concentration of >200 mg/dL during a glucose tolerance test.

A. This value is incorrect. See explanation for B.

C. A 2-hour plasma glucose tolerance test may be used when a patient does not have a fasting blood sugar >126 mg/dL, but there is still concern for diabetes. An oral glucose load of 75 g is given to the patient, and blood sugar is measured at 1 and 2 hours. A blood sugar >140 mg/dL and <200 mg/dL at the 2-hour mark constitutes "glucose intolerance," but not frank diabetes. These patients are at risk for the development of overt diabetes and should be monitored carefully.

D. Hemoglobin A1C, or glycosylated hemoglobin, is currently not used as a diagnostic criterion for diabetes, because standardization of these tests is lacking between laboratories. Variation in A1C numbers can also be seen in various states of anemia (iron deficiency, hemolysis) and in end-stage renal disease.

E. Ketosis and an anion gap acidosis do not diagnose diabetes. It may be due to alcoholism or starvation as well as insulin deficiency states and is differentiated from diabetic ketoacidosis by the normal or low blood sugar seen in this entity. There is also a higher ratio of acetoacetate to beta-hydroxybutyrate seen in alcoholic or starvation ketoacidosis versus diabetic ketoacidosis.

163. **B.** MRI is the preferred imaging test to evaluate a patient for a prolactinoma. Prolactinomas are the most common pituitary tumor, and present in women with symptoms of oligomenorrhea, amenorrhea, and galactorrhea. Microadenomas are lesions <1 cm, and macroadenomas are >1 cm.

A. CT of the head is not the first-line choice in patients with elevated prolactin levels and symptoms of hyperprolactinemia; MRI can better evaluate the hypothalamic/pituitary stalk for masses.

C. Plain skull films are not sensitive enough to evaluate for a hypothalamic/pituitary mass.

D. It is always essential to search for other causes of high prolactin levels, such as hypothyroidism, dopamine-antagonist drugs such as antiemetics and antipsychotics, and pregnancy. Usually, however, a patient with a prolactin level >300 ng/mL will have a prolactin-secreting tumor.

E. Dopamine agonists such as bromocriptine decrease the prolactin level whether the cause of elevated prolactin is a prolactin-secreting tumor or there is a secondary cause. Therefore, it is not helpful to use bromocriptine to diagnose a prolactinoma. Bromocriptine is the primary therapy for prolactinomas. Side effects include nausea, vomiting, and orthostatic hypotension, which can make it hard to tolerate. Some patients who cannot tolerate the GI side effects can use an intravaginal preparation, which is better tolerated.

164. **E.** Symptoms of hyperthyroidism include palpitations, diarrhea, tremulousness, unintentional weight loss, heat intolerance, and hair thinning. Graves' disease is the most common cause of hyperthyroidism and typically occurs in women between the ages of 20 and 40 years old. Clinical findings of Graves' disease include hyperthyroidism with a diffuse, nontender goiter; ophthalmopathy (to include lid lag, lid retraction, proptosis, extraocular muscle weakness); and pretibial myxedema. Patients do not need all three components to have Graves'. The diagnosis is made by finding a decreased thyroid stimulating hormone, an elevated thyroxine level and an increased radioactive iodide uptake value. Multiple options are available for treatment of Graves' disease: Surgical removal or radioactive iodine ablation of the gland will permanently alter the gland, and many patients become hypothyroid either immediately or over time. Medical therapies to block hormone synthesis with methimazole or propylthiouracil are other alternatives.

A. Subacute thyroiditis, also called de Quervain's thyroiditis, is probably virally mediated. Other forms of thyroiditis include chronic and postpartum forms. In thyroiditis, a transient thyrotoxicosis exists secondary to leakage of hormone from the gland, then transient hypothyroidism, then a return of thyroid function to normal. Radioactive iodide uptake scan, which is ordered to evaluate the cause of the clinical hyperthyroidism, usually shows a low uptake due to injury or inflammation of the gland.

C. Addison's disease is the name for primary adrenal insufficiency. Symptoms include weakness, anorexia, vomiting, diffuse abdominal pain, and hypotension. The diagnosis is made by doing a corticotropin stimulation test. This involves obtaining a baseline cortisol level and then giving the patient a dose of adrenal corticotropin hormone (ACTH) to try to stimulate the adrenal glands. A cortisol level is obtained at 30, 60, and 90 minutes after the ACTH is given. The cortisol level should rise appropriately to indicate that the adrenals are able to function appropriately when stimulated. This patient does not have Addison's disease.

D. Hashimoto's thyroiditis is a clinical state of hypothyroidism. It is usually seen in women aged 20 to 60 years and may be secondary to autoimmune destruction with lymphocytic infiltration of the thyroid gland. Thyroid-stimulating hormone is usually elevated and patients present with symptoms of hypothyroidism including fatigue, depression, cold intolerance, and weight gain. Treatment is with thyroid hormone replacement.

---

165. **C.** This patient likely has primary adrenal insufficiency or Addison's disease. Symptoms include weakness, lethargy, and fatigue as well as nausea, vomiting, abdominal pain, headaches, and weight loss. The adrenal glands produce cortisol, mineralocorticoids, and sex hormones. Deficiency of mineralocorticoids such as aldosterone causes the hyponatremia and hyperkalemia that are the hallmark electrolyte disturbances of primary adrenal insufficiency. Patients may be somewhat hypoglycemic due to cortisol deficiency. The patient's skin pigmentation is due to overproduction of ACTH-pro-opiate melanocorticotropin (POMC) from the hypothalamus/pituitary that is an attempt to stimulate the failing glands. The precursor hormone of ACTH is ACTH-POMC. POMC is cleaved from ACTH and stimulates melanocytes to produce melanin. Lastly, eosinophilia is sometimes seen in primary adrenal insufficiency. In the United States, primary adrenal insufficiency is most often due to an autoimmune destruction of the gland.

A. Patients with hyperthyroidism also experience weight loss, anxiety, and tremulousness, but they should not have the hyperpigmentation or the electrolyte disturbances that are seen in primary adrenal insufficiency.

B. Hypothyroidism gives a clinical picture of fatigue, sluggishness, and lethargy. Patients will also complain of weight gain, constipation, and cold intolerance. They will not have skin color changes or electrolyte abnormalities.

D. Secondary hypoadrenalism is a lesion of the pituitary and presents with symptoms similar to primary hypoadrenalism, with the exception of hyperkalemia and increased pigmentation. In these patients, ACTH levels are low. Remember that aldosterone is released from the adrenal gland because of the stimulation of the renin-angiotensin system and *not* because of the stimulation of ACTH. This is why, in secondary adrenal insufficiency, the potassium is usually normal. (Glucocorticoids affect water/sodium balance, allowing patients with secondary hypoadrenalism to have some degree of hyponatremia.)

E. Hyperaldosteronism usually manifests itself as hypertension and hypokalemia. This patient is hypotensive and hyperkalemic, more suggestive of someone with relative hypoaldosteronism, effects of which can be seen with primary adrenal insufficiency.

166. **B.** Polycystic ovarian syndrome is a constellation of oligo-ovulation, hyperandrogenism, and ovarian cysts. Hirsutism is secondary to increased levels of androgens.

A. Idiopathic hirsutism is associated with regular ovulatory cycles and no other medical problems. It may be related to ethnicity, and some people from Mediterranean populations are especially hairy. The most important question to ask a woman who presents with complaints of hirsutism is whether her menses are regular or not. If she says that her menses are extremely regular, then there is no further work-up to do. Patients may be referred to dermatologists or cosmetologists for hair removal.

C. Pituitary neoplasms, such as prolactinomas, can cause irregular periods but usually cause other symptoms such as headache, visual changes (depending on tumor size), and galactorrhea. Prolactinomas are not associated with hirsutism.

D. Medications can cause hirsutism, but phenobarbital is not one of these medications. Phenytoin, glucocorticoids, and pencillamine are known to cause increased hair growth.

E. Hypothyroidism can cause irregular periods and changes in hair growth (more coarse), but this patient has normal TSH and thyroxine levels.

167. **C.** This patient's hypercalcemia is likely secondary to malignancy, especially given his history of weight loss, smoking, and physical exam findings. Malignancy can cause hypercalcemia by many different paraneoplastic syndromes. Solid tumors such as squamous cell carcinoma and renal cell carcinoma often secrete parathyroid hormone-related peptide (PTH-rP) that stimulates the release of calcium from bone into the circulation. Breast cancer and melanoma cause hypercalcemia because of the direct invasion of bone. Lymphomas often cause an increase in calcium secondary to an increase in the amount of 1,25 hydroxyvitamin D.

A. Primary hyperparathyroidism causes elevated calcium by secretion of PTH. Parathyroid adenomas account for 80% of these cases, and parathyroid hyperplasia accounts for 15% to 20% of primary hyperparathyroidism. The diagnosis is often made by incidental laboratory findings of mildly elevated calcium levels. When work-up is done to evaluate the cause of the hypercalcemia, the intact PTH is found to be elevated inappropriately for the calcium level. (Normally, hypercalcemia should suppress intact PTH.)

B. Vitamin D excess can cause hypercalcemia. Vitamin D levels may become elevated, resulting in hypercalcemia, secondary to granulomatous disease such as sarcoidosis, coccidioidomycosis, histoplasmosis, and tuberculosis.

D. Various medications can cause hypercalcemia. β-blockers are not common contributors. Thiazides, lithium, vitamin A, and calcium-containing antacids are known to cause hypercalcemia.

E. Hyperthyroidism can cause hypercalcemia secondary to increased bone turnover. Immobilization and Paget's disease also cause hypercalcemia by the same mechanism. This patient's history and physical exam do not suggest elevated thyroid hormone levels.

168. | **B.** A C-peptide level would help determine the difference between endogenous and exogenous insulin administration. If this patient had surreptitiously injected insulin, her C-peptide level should be low. C-peptide is a portion of the proinsulin produced endogenously.

A. An elevated insulin level would be suggest either an endogenous source of insulin such as an insulinoma or exogenous insulin levels. It cannot distinguish between the two.

C. A sulfonylurea level would help determine if the patient had ingested sulfonylurea. This patient has no contact with anyone taking oral hypoglycemics, so this is unlikely.

D. Elevated liver enzymes can suggest a toxic (e.g., acetaminophen overdose), shock, or viral insult to the liver that cause hypoglycemia. This patient denies any Tylenol use and has no history of chronic alcohol use, which could also cause hypoglycemia.

E. Hypothyroidism may rarely cause hypoglycemia, but this patient has no evidence of hypothyroidism on physical exam.

169. | **E.** This patient has hypercalcemia manifesting as mental status changes and abdominal and bone pain. A possible etiology is her thiazide diuretic use, but regardless of the etiology, patients with hypercalcemia have undergone an osmotic diuresis due to the high calcium's effect on the kidneys and are significantly volume depleted. A normal saline bolus, even upwards of 4 to 6 liters, is required to lower her serum calcium levels before any other intervention, such as Lasix. Giving fluids is the first step in treating a patient with symptomatic hypercalcemia.

A. Glucocorticoids are useful in treating hypercalcemia that is related to high levels of vitamin D, such as the hypercalcemia found in sarcoidosis and certain lymphomas. The calcium level improves within days, and mechanism of action is unknown.

B. Furosemide, along with normal saline, is also one of the first steps in treating symptomatic hypercalcemia. It is only started after a patient is intravascularly repleted. Like normal saline, it promotes natriuresis and therefore increases calcium excretion.

C. Bisphosphonates inhibit osteoclast function. Osteoclasts resorb bone, which releases calcium into the circulation; therefore, bisphosphonates inhibit the release of calcium. They are very useful in treating the hypercalcemia of malignancy. Onset of action is 1 to 2 days, and duration of therapy is up to 2 weeks.

D. Calcitonin simulates the endogenous hormone that is produced by the parathyroid glands and that aids in putting serum calcium into bone. Onset is within hours, and duration of effect is 2 to 3 days. Unfortunately, a major side effect is tachyphylaxis.

170. | **A.** Fibrates decrease secretion of VLDL and increase stimulation of lipoprotein lipase, which in turn leads to increased clearance of triglycerides. Fibrates are used primarily to reduce elevated triglycerides, but also may increase serum HDL.

B. Statins are inhibitors of hydroxy-methylglutaryl-coenzyme A (HMG-CoA) reductase, which is the rate-limiting step in cholesterol synthesis. Inhibition of this reductase leads to increased LDL receptor turnover, thus leading to decreases in serum LDL. Statins are the most effective medication for reducing LDL levels. Side effects include hepatitis and myopathy and are more common in patients who are on both statins and fibrates. Therefore, it is very important to educate patients about the side effects.

C. Niacin inhibits production of VLDL and, in turn, LDL. It also reduces transfer of HDL to VLDL, thereby increasing serum HDL levels. Niacin is used in patients to lower LDL, increase HDL, and decrease triglycerides. Side effects include flushing, pruritus, and insulin resistance.

D. Bile acid sequestrants such as cholestyramine inhibit bile acid reabsorption, which leads to a decreased pool of cholesterol. This in turn increases the number of LDL receptors, which lowers serum LDL levels. These medications primarily work to lower LDL levels. Side effects include abdominal distension and change in bowel habits.

E. Cholesterol absorption inhibitors are a relatively new class of medications that inhibit the absorption of cholesterol at the intestinal brush border without affecting the absorption of fat-soluble vitamins. This treatment is currently thought to be adjunctive therapy to statins in lowering serum LDL levels. Side effects include hepatitis, so liver function tests should be followed.

171. **E.** Vitamin D deficiency can be caused by decreased intake, inadequate production in the skin, or renal failure. In renal failure there is decreased hydroxylation of calcidiol to calcitriol, the end product of vitamin D. The function of vitamin D is to increase absorption of calcium and phosphate at the level of the intestine. Deficiency causes reduced absorption of both calcium and phosphate, which leads to increased production of PTH (secondary hyperparathyroidism) as an attempt to improve serum calcium levels, which then lowers serum phosphate levels.

172. **B.** Hypercalcemia of malignancy can be secondary to production of a PTH-related protein or local osteoclastic activity at the level of bone. Calcium levels are elevated and phosphate levels can vary depending on the etiology of the elevated calcium. Endogenous PTH levels will be low in response to feedback inhibition from the elevated serum calcium.

173. **C.** Hypoparathyroidism can be isolated, secondary to surgery, or due to decreased magnesium levels. PTH is responsible for increasing serum calcium from bone, increasing serum calcium resorption at the level of the kidney, and decreasing serum phosphate levels by excretion by the kidney. Thus, in hypoparathyroidism, calcium levels should be low and phosphate levels should be elevated.

174. **D.** Pseudohypoparathyroidism is defined as PTH end-organ resistance. This syndrome is also associated with skeletal abnormalities and retardation. Consequently, serum calcium levels are low, serum phosphate levels are elevated, and serum PTH levels are elevated.

175. **A.** Hyperparathyroidism is caused by an adenoma 80% of the time. It can also be caused by hyperplasia and carcinoma. With too much PTH, there is increased serum concentration of calcium from bony turnover and increased renal absorption of calcium. Phosphate excretion is increased at the level of the kidney.

176. **C.** Many medications can lead to impotence. Of the antihypertensive medications, thiazides and β-blockers have potential side effects of impotence. Most antidepressants, some H2 blockers, and antifungal drugs can also cause impotence.

A. People with spinal cord injuries can develop erectile dysfunction. Patients with neurogenic causes of impotence such as spinal cord injury are unable to have erections while sleeping and should not have the cremasteric reflex.

B. Any patient with evidence of peripheral vascular disease can develop impotence. Like patients with neurogenic causes of impotence, however, they are do not have erections during REM sleep.

D. Depression and anxiety are major causes of impotence. Sudden loss of an erection, or inability to maintain an erection, is a common sign. These patients can maintain an erection at night while sleeping.

E. Hypogonadism is a common problem plaguing older men. Decreased libido and impotence are common manifestations. Testosterone replacement is the treatment. This patient is unlikely to have this problem, because he does not have testicular atrophy.

177. **A.** This patient has anti-phospholipid antibody syndrome. Patients with this syndrome have antibodies directed toward certain phospholipid-bound plasma proteins that are involved in the coagulation pathway. Patients are predisposed to recurrent arterial and venous clot formation and fetal loss. Laboratory testing includes lupus anticoagulant. The patient's serum is mixed with normal patient serum to see whether the aPTT corrects. If it does not, the test is positive for an inhibitor, most likely the lupus anticoagulant. Thrombocytopenia is also associated with this syndrome. PT is not affected.

178. **E.** Hemophilia B is an X-linked inherited bleeding disorder. Patients usually present with prolonged bleeding, hematomas, or hemarthrosis. Factor IX is deficient in hemophilia B, and factor VIII is deficient in hemophilia A.

179. **C.** Von Willebrand's disease is the most common inherited bleeding disorder. Patients usually have easy bruising, nosebleeds, menorrhagia, or prolonged bleeding with trauma. Von Willebrand factor plays a critical role in platelet function and is also a carrier protein for factor VIII. Defective von Willebrand factor can therefore decrease factor VIII and prolong PTT.

180. **B.** DIC is triggered by systemic illness and can be a catastrophic hematologic event. Possible associations with DIC include sepsis, trauma, malignancy, and burns. Initially, fibrinogen and platelets are consumed in clot formation. This is later followed by hemorrhage as the clots are degraded by fibrinolysis.

181. **B.** Primary hyperparathyroidism occurs in women three times more often than men, and it is usually seen in the early postmenopausal years. It is most commonly asymptomatic and is diagnosed because a mildly elevated calcium level is seen on blood that is being tested for some other reason. Patients have an elevated PTH, and in 80% of cases it is due to a parathyroid adenoma. Approximately 20% of the time, the elevated PTH is due to diffuse parathyroid gland hyperplasia.

182. **C.** Familial hypocalciuric hypercalcemia (FHH) is an autosomal dominant trait that consists of moderate hypercalcemia (usually asymptomatic) and a relative hypocalciuria. The renal tubular resorption of calcium and magnesium is abnormally high. The *best* test to determine whether or not a patient has FHH is *not* a 24 hour total calcium excretion level, but rather a ratio of calcium clearance to creatinine clearance. The clearance ratio in FHH is one-third that of primary hyperparathyroidism, with a cutoff value at 0.01. This test helps to distinguish FHH from primary hyperparathyroidism.

183. **E.** PTH-rP is a protein that is released in excess in certain malignancy states. It mimics PTH and binds its receptor with equal affinity. It causes a humoral hypercalcemia of malignancy, and is most often seen in squamous cancers of the head and neck and of the lung. PTH-rP activates osteoclasts to resorb bone and release calcium. Intact PTH (iPTH) is suppressed in the hypercalcemia that is related to PTH-rP excess.

184. **D.** Hypercalcemia secondary to granulomatous diseases, such as sarcoidosis, is mediated by an abnormally elevated 1,25-dihydroxyvitamin D level. The conversion of hydroxyvitamin D to dihydroxyvitamin D appears to be unregulated in these patients, and is suppressed by glucocorticoids, which is the appropriate treatment.

185. | **A.** Hypercalcemia occurs in 20% to 40% of patients with multiple myeloma during their disease course. Myeloma cells in the bone marrow produce cytokines that activate the nearby osteoclasts to resorb bone. Interestingly, there is not a close correlation between the amount of bony destruction and bone pain in myeloma and the development of hypercalcemia.

186. | **D.** Often used by men to relieve symptoms of BPH, saw palmetto is thought to inhibit 5-α reductase type I or androgen receptor activity. It is associated with few adverse side effects.

187. | **E.** Used in the treatment of mild to moderate depression, St. John's wort has ten active ingredients, effects of which are unclear.

188. | **A.** Ginkgo biloba is used primarily in the treatment of dementia and claudication. Adverse side effects include headache and intestinal discomfort.

189. | **B.** Derived from the purple coneflower, echinacea is used to fight the common cold or respiratory viruses. No significant side effects are noted.

190. | **C.** Although no data are available regarding its safety, ginseng is used by many to combat fatigue.

191. | **A.** LDL cholesterol goals are based on number of risk factors for coronary artery disease (CAD). Patients with one risk factor initiate diet control at levels >160 mg/dL and drug therapy at levels >190 mg/dL, and the goal is <160 mg/dL. Patients with two risk factors for CAD initiate diet control at levels >130 mg/dL and drug therapy at levels >160 mg/dL, and the goal is <130 mg/dL. Risk factors include age >45 in men and >55 in women, tobacco use, hypertension, diabetes, family history, and HDL <35 mg/dL. This patient has two risk factors (age and medically controlled hypertension), thus it would be recommended to start statins for a goal LDL of <130 mg/dL.

192. | **B.** This patient has one risk factor for CAD: her family history. At this point, her therapy should consist of lifestyle changes, with a goal of LDL <160 mg/dL.

193. | **A.** This patient has a history of CAD. Her LDL goal should be <100 mg/dL. Statins are added once LDL reaches 130 mg/dL, and are considered when LDL is between 100 and 130 mg/dL.

194. **B.** Vitamin A deficiency occurs mainly in the third world and is due to dietary deficiency of the vitamin. The main manifestations of vitamin A deficiency are related to the eye, and vitamin A deficiency is a leading cause of blindness in the third world. Skin manifestations that may occur consist of hyperkeratosis of the epidermis, especially the follicular area. This results in a perifollicular hyperkeratosis called phrynoderma or "toad skin."

195. **E.** Deficiency of niacin causes pellagra, the symptoms of which are commonly referred to as the "three Ds": diarrhea, dementia, and dermatitis. The dermatitis may manifest in several ways but usually consists of erythema of the dorsa of the hands (due to the distribution in sun-exposed areas), which progresses to blisters, then bullae. These lesions are pathognomonic for niacin deficiency.

196. **F.** Riboflavin deficiency may result in several dermal manifestations, such as angular stomatitis, glossitis, and conjunctivitis.

197. **C.** Vitamin B_{12} deficiency is known to cause megaloblastic anemia, nail changes, and beefy red tongue. Skin manifestations consist of hypopigmented macules that tend to be distributed on flexural areas of skin.

198. **A.** Vitamin C deficiency is uncommon in developed countries. It causes scurvy, a syndrome characterized by myalgias, malaise, and weakness; perifollicular purpura follow, primarily on the legs. Hemarthroses may also occur, resulting in significant pain.

199. **G.** Vitamin B_6 deficiency may result from treatment with isoniazid or other medications without supplementation of pyridoxine. It may also result from dietary deficiency. It results in constitutional symptoms and neurologic disturbances. Skin findings in pyridoxine deficiency include seborrhea involving the face, scalp, neck, shoulders, buttocks, and perineum.

D. Alopecia is defined as an absence of hair from areas where it normally grows. It may be due to hormones, as in male-pattern baldness; to infections, as in tinea capitis; or to autoimmune diseases, as in alopecia areata or alopecia totalis. There are no vitamin deficiencies that cause alopecia.

200. | **B.** This patient has type II diabetes mellitus that is confirmed by two separate fasting glucose measurements >126. He is obese and has significant insulin resistance based on the physical exam finding of acanthosis nigricans. This patient also appears to have the "metabolic syndrome" with his hypertension, diabetes, and obesity, and should have his lipids evaluated. It is reasonable to encourage diet and exercise therapies, but it is unlikely that this approach alone will change the metabolic profile in this patient, unless he is extremely motivated. Therefore, the first choice of pharmacotherapy is metformin. This is the only oral agent used for the treatment of diabetes type II that does not cause weight gain in overweight patients and that does not cause hypoglycemia in patients whose fasting blood sugar is less than 150 mg/dL. Therefore, it is the optimal choice in this patient.

A. Diet and exercise should be encouraged. The patient should have a thorough cardiac evaluation before beginning an exercise program because of the significant cardiac risks of diabetes and hypertension (and probable hyperlipidemia). Diet and exercise alone, however, are not likely to change the metabolic picture, and it is reasonable to start pharmacologic therapy.

C. Sulfonylureas are often chosen first-line in diabetes management; however, it is not a good choice in this patient for two reasons. First, it can cause weight gain, and this patient is already obese (BMI >30). Second, sulfonylureas can cause hypoglycemia as a side effect, and should not be used to start therapy in patients whose fasting blood sugar is ≤150 mg/dL. They also should be used with caution in patients who are elderly or who have renal insufficiency.

D. All type II diabetics who live long enough will eventually require insulin as the β-cell function of the pancreas fails. However, this patient still has good function with a fasting blood sugar of 150 or so, and should not require insulin at this point.

E. The diagnosis of diabetes is made by the fasting blood sugar measurements. There is no need to "confirm" the diagnosis with a hemoglobin A1C measurement. Even if the A1C were normal, he would still have the diagnosis of diabetes based on the fasting sugars.

Index

Index note: page references with an *f* or a *t* indicate a figure or table on designated page; page references in **bold** indicate discussion of the subject in the Answers and Explanations sections.

DREXEL UNIVERSITY
HEALTH SCIENCES LIBRARIES
HAHNEMANN LIBRARY